An Atlas of
BREAST DISEASE

THE ENCYCLOPEDIA OF VISUAL MEDICINE SERIES

An Atlas of
BREAST DISEASE

James A. Hall, MD, FACOG, FACS

Obstetrician/Gynecologist, Women's Health Center of Logansport; and
Clinical Associate Professor, Department of Obstetrics and Gynecology
Indiana University, Indianapolis, Indiana

and

John V. Knaus, DO, FACOG, FACS

Chairman, Department of Obstetrics and Gynecology
Director of Gynecologic Oncology
Director of Obstetrics and Gynecology Residency Program
Saint Francis Hospital, Evanston; and
Clinical Professor, Department of Obstetrics and Gynecology
University of Illinois at Chicago, Chicago, Illinois

The Parthenon Publishing Group
International Publishers in Medicine, Science & Technology

A CRC PRESS COMPANY
BOCA RATON   LONDON   NEW YORK   WASHINGTON, D.C.

Published in the USA by
The Parthenon Publishing Group
345 Park Avenue South
New York, NY 10010, USA

Published in the UK by
The Parthenon Publishing Group
23–25 Blades Court
Deodar Road
London, SW15 2NU, UK

Library of Congress Cataloging-in-Publication Data
Hall, James A. (James Alan), 1949-
    An atlas of breast disease/James A. Hall and John V. Knaus.
        p. ; cm. -- (The encyclopedia of visual medicine series)
    Includes bibliographical references and index.
    ISBN 1-85070-533-X (alk. paper)
    1. Breast–Diseases--Atlases. 2. Breast--Diseases--Diagnosis--Atlases. 3. Breast--Radiography--
    Atlases. 4. Diagnosis, Radioscopic--Atlases. I. Knaus, John V. II. Title. III. Series.
        [DNLM: 1. Breast Diseases--Atlases. 2. Mammography--Atlases. WP 17 H177a2003]
    RG492.H35 2003
    618.1'9'00222--dc21

                                                                        2003040561

British Library Cataloguing in Publication Data
Hall, James A.
    An atlas of breast disease. - (The encyclopedia of visual medicine series)
    1. Breast - Diseases 2. Breast - Diseases - Diagnosis
    I. Title II. Knaus, John V.
    618.1'9

ISBN 1-85070-533X

Composition by The Parthenon Publishing Group, London, UK
Color reproduction by Graphic Reproductions, Morecambe, UK
Printed and bound by T. G. Hostench S. A., Spain

Contents

Dedication

Bill Hindle, MD, has encouraged my participation in medical education and has been my mentor. Bill has been instrumental in and an advocate for the improvement of breast care for women. He and I both feel the importance of the primary care physician and the need to eliminate traditional turf wars.

All I do is for my wife Kyle and kids Audrey, Courtney, Lynly, and Cassie. They are my inspiration and link to a faith-filled life. This book and my life are dedicated to them.

No dedication would be complete without mentioning my dad, Bernard R. Hall, MD, a hard working Obstetrician–Gynecologist (now retired) from the old school. He was ahead of his time with a belief that breast care belonged as a routine part of gynecology. His breast knowledge and surgical expertise became the foundation of my interest and education in breast care. I will be forever grateful and appreciative of the opportunity I have had with him as my practice partner, mentor, and father.

James A. Hall MD, FACOG, FACS

In 1977, I met John H. Isaacs, MD. From that day in April, when he interviewed me as an Obstetrics and Gynecology Resident candidate, through his Fellowship in Gynecologic Oncology and as private practitioners together, Dr Isaacs has profoundly affected and guided my professional career. Everyone should have the benefit of such a mentor and role model.

Personally, I dedicate this book to the three true loves of my life – my wife, Laura and my two daughters, Jennifer and Sarah.

On a daily basis, the patients I am privileged to care for amaze me with their stamina and faith. I remain indebted to them.

John V. Knaus DO, FACOG, FACS

Preface

An Atlas of Breast Disease is a practical guide for the primary care clinician. The evaluation and management of a breast complaint is often the responsibility of the patient's primary care physician and, with proper information, most problems can be evaluated and treated in the office setting without referral. It is important to understand the inseparable relationship between breast health and overall women's health care. We have written this text to illustrate 'how we do it' in an easy-to-learn format. We hope the reader finds it to be of value in the healthcare needs of women.

James A. Hall MD, FACOG, FACS
John V. Knaus DO, FACOG, FACS

Acknowledgements

I have been privileged and honored to be able to provide total breast care to the women served by the Women's Health Center of Logansport. No one functions as an island and I am blessed with talented and supportive practice partners, Duffy Murphy, MD, and Jeffrey VanCuren, MD. My co-author John Knaus is a good friend and mentor. Our patients constantly amaze us with their courage, loyalty and dedication to what is right.

Cancer is an evil enemy robbing patients and families out of more than life. Fear of recurrence and side-effects from treatment are thieves that forever lurk in the distance of cancer patients. Lives are changed forever and the journey is a long, rough road. Optimism, faith, trust, friends, and family support are the foundation of a successful cancer journey in association with early diagnosis and appropriate treatment. Two patients come to mind as being, each in their own way, role models for this journey: our good friend and patient Beth Workman has successfully battled breast cancer, and our good friend Brandt Ludlow, MD, successfully defeated head and neck cancer. Both should be acknowledged for how they live their lives without surrender to disease. They are an inspiration to all who know them.

My sincere thanks to the Parthenon Publishing Group, especially Nat Russo who started this project and Dinah Alam who provided the 'gentle' motivation for its completion.

James A. Hall MD, FACOG, FACS

This text represents the combined efforts of several individuals. Nat Russo initiated the project over lunch with Dr James Hall and I several years ago in Philadelphia. More recently, Dinah Alam has provided the momentum to complete the project. My co-author and good friend, Jim Hall always met the deadlines – I never did!

I wish to thank Dr Marko Jachtorowycz, my practice partner and close friend (a rare and valuable combination), Dr Janis Atkinson (pathologist extraordinaire) for her photomicrograph assistance, Shirley Miller RN, for years of dedicated support, and Constance Clarke, my secretary and antidote for completion-anxiety during the final hectic days of the text's completion.

John V. Knaus, DO, FACOG, FACS

Foreword

Most women fear breast cancer. Primary health care providers for women, including Obstetrician–Gynecologists, can serve as a readily available source of current, accurate information about the management of breast cancer, as well as benign breast problems. What is needed is a clear, concise, state-of-the-art resource for clinicians to consult about breast care, diagnosis and treatment. Drs James Hall and John Knaus have ably filled this need with their book *An Atlas of Breast Disease*.

The Atlas, with its abundant and succinct colored algorithms, charts, graphs, and figures, presents complex information in brief, lucid, and easily understandable formats that can be quickly grasped by the reader. Numerous tables, illustrative mammograms, and 'key points' summaries, drawn from the authors' clinical practice and extensive experience, complement the readily readable, clinically oriented text. Color photomicrographs of pertinent typical histology and pathology amply add visual impact to the related text. Throughout, the artwork is exceptionally clear and clean with evident clinical significance.

Furthermore, this useful Atlas can be recommended to students and patients with an interest in breast disease and particularly breast cancer. Any reader would not only benefit from an initial careful reading of the Atlas, but could also use it as a practical refresher and clinical reference. Eventually, in clinical practice, patients will surely benefit from the material that is so clearly presented in this Atlas.

I enjoyed reading the Atlas and was keenly impressed with the format and artwork. Drs Hall and Knaus are to be highly commended for sharing their clinical insights and experience in such an easily accessed volume.

William H. Hindle MD, FACOG, FACS

Professor Emeritus
Department of Obstetrics and Gynecology
Keck School of Medicine
University of Southern California;
and
Founder, Breast Diagnostic Center
Women's and Children's Hospital
LAC and USC Medical Center
Los Angeles, California

CHAPTER 1

Role of the primary care physician

Breast cancer is the most common malignancy found among women in the United States and only lung cancer has a higher mortality rate. Breast cancer annual incidence is nearly twice that of any other female adult cancer and accounts for nearly one-third of all newly diagnosed cancers in women. The American Cancer Society estimates that there were 211 300 new cases of invasive breast cancer in 2002 and 39 800 deaths (Tables 1.1 and 1.2)[1]. A complete listing of United States breast cancer cases and deaths is shown in Table 1.3[2]. The incidence of *in situ* disease has increased since the widespread use of mammogram screening programs.

One in eight women living to 95 years of age will develop breast cancer in her lifetime (Table 1.4)[3] and breast cancer is the leading cause of death of women in their 40s. Breast cancer incidence increases with age until the risk plateaus in the 70s (Table 1.5)[4]. On the whole, primary care physicians will discover more breast cancers than any other malignancy. Benign breast problems are also a frequent cause of women seeking health care.

The primary care physician has a responsibility to not only provide screening for the asymptomatic patient but also to fully investigate a breast complaint. Nearly all problems can be investigated thoroughly in the office setting and rarely require

Table 1.1 Estimated numbers of new cancer cases in women: United States, 2002. Data from reference 1

Site	Number of cases	Percentage of total cases of cancer
Breast	211 300	32
Lung/bronchus	80 100	12
Colon/rectum	74 700	11
Uterine corpus	40 100	6
Ovary	25 400	4
Remainder of sites	227 200	35

Table 1.2 Estimated number of deaths from cancer in women: United States, 2002. Data from reference 1

Site	Number of deaths	Percentage of total deaths from cancer
Lung/bronchus	68 800	25
Breast	39 800	15
Colon/rectum	28 800	11
Pancreas	15 300	6
Ovary	14 300	5
Remainder of sites	103 600	34

referral. Although most complaints result from benign etiologies, it is the fear of cancer that motivates most women to seek healthcare. Breast cancer is a highly curable disease when discovered

Table 1.3 Estimated new breast cancer cases and deaths in women by age, United States, 2001–2002. Table reproduced with permission from reference 2

Age	In situ cases		Invasive cases		Deaths	
	(n)	(%)	(n)	(%)	(n)	(%)
<30	100	0.2	900	0.5	100	0.2
30–39	1600	3.4	8000	4.2	1200	3.0
40–49	10800	22.9	35400	18.4	5000	12.5
50–59	12500	26.5	46800	24.3	7300	18.3
60–69	9400	19.9	33100	17.2	5900	14.6
70–79	9400	19.9	43000	22.4	9800	24.3
80+	3300	7.0	25000	13.0	10900	27.2
Total	47100	100.0	192200	100.0	40200	100.0

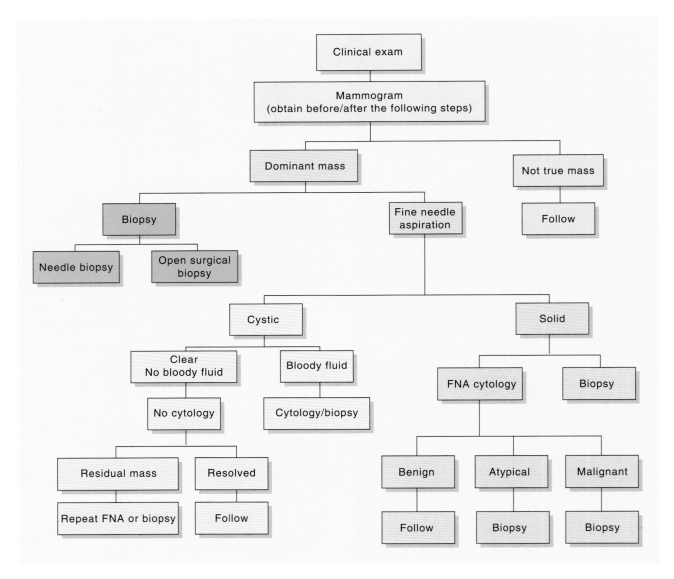

Figure 1.1 Algorithm for clinical investigation of a palpable breast mass

Table 1.4 Accumulated lifetime risk of developing breast cancer for a 20-year-old woman. Data from reference 3

Age (years)	Risk
25	1/19608
30	1/2525
35	1/622
40	1/217
45	1/93
50	1/50
55	1/33
60	1/24
65	1/17
70	1/14
75	1/11
80	1/10
85	1/9
Lifetime	1/8

Table 1.5 Increasing breast cancer risk with age. Data from reference 4

Age	Cancers/100000 women/year
25–29	7.4
30–34	26.7
35–39	66.2
40–44	129.4
45–49	159.4
50–54	220.0
55–59	261.6
60–64	330.7
65–69	390.7
70–74	421.8
75–79	461.4
80–84	451.3
85+	411.9

early. Non-palpable tumors discovered by mammography are curable at least 90% of the time, as opposed to palpable tumors of which at least 50% have metastatic spread to lymphatics.

The value of breast self-examination is limited to the earlier diagnosis of palpable tumors than would have been discovered at the next routine physical exam. Although breast self-examination has not been shown to reduce overall breast cancer mortality, it should be recommended so tumors can be discovered as early as possible in each individual patient. Delayed diagnosis of breast cancer has become a frequent cause of medical malpractice litigation in the USA. Recommendation of mammography screening protocols, prompt investigation of abnormalities, appropriate referral and accurate charting are the foundations of malpractice defense.

The diagnostic triad of clinical breast examination, mammography, and fine needle aspiration will accurately diagnose nearly all breast complaints (Figures 1.1 and 1.2). Ultrasound is an adjunct to mammography and has limited use for screening. It is essential that there is concordance of all results from the diagnostic triad. Any variation from total agreement of results requires further investigation.

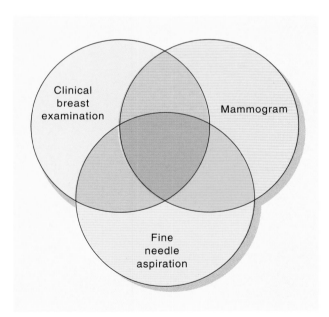

Figure 1.2 The diagnostic triad consists of clinical breast examination, mammography, and fine needle aspiration. Concordance of results will nearly always lead to the correct diagnosis in the office setting. Disagreement among findings requires further investigation

REFERENCES

1. American Cancer Society, Inc. *Cancer Facts and Figures 2003*. Atlanta: ACS, 2003. Available at http://www.cancer.org/docroot/STT/stt_0.asp. March 2003

2. American Cancer Society, Inc. *Breast Cancer Facts and Figures 2001–2002*. Atlanta: ACS, 2003. Available at http://www.cancer.org/docroot/STT/content/STT_1x_Breast_Cancer_Facts_and_Figures_2001-2002.asp. Viewed March 2003

3. Feuer EJ, Wun L-M, Boring CC, *et al.* The lifetime risk of developing breast cancer. *J Natl Cancer Inst* 1993; 85:892–7

4. National Cancer Institute. *SEER Data 1984–1988. National Institutes of Health National Cancer Institute Statistics Review 1975–1988.* Bethesda, MD: National Institutes of Health; 1991: NIH Publication no. 91–2789

KEY POINTS: ROLE OF PRIMARY CARE

1. Breast complaints result from benign conditions far more commonly than from malignant conditions

2. Breast cancer is the most common cancer found in women and the second most frequent cause of cancer death

3. The presence or absence of risk factors should not influence the evaluation of a breast complaint as all women are at risk for cancer

4. Early detection is the most important factor in breast cancer survival

5. Every breast complaint should be fully evaluated until the diagnosis is secure

CHAPTER 2

Anatomy of the breast

The breasts are modified sebaceous glands within the superficial fascia of the anterior chest wall. The average adult breast weighs 200–300 grams and is composed of 80% fat and connective tissue and 20% glandular tissue. Figure 2.1 illustrates the cross-sectional anatomy of the breast and

Figure 2.2 shows the terms used to describe the anatomic divisions of the breast.

The lateral projection is called the Tail of Spence and expands in the upper-outer direction towards the axilla. The breast is composed of 15–20 lobes arranged in a radial fashion extending

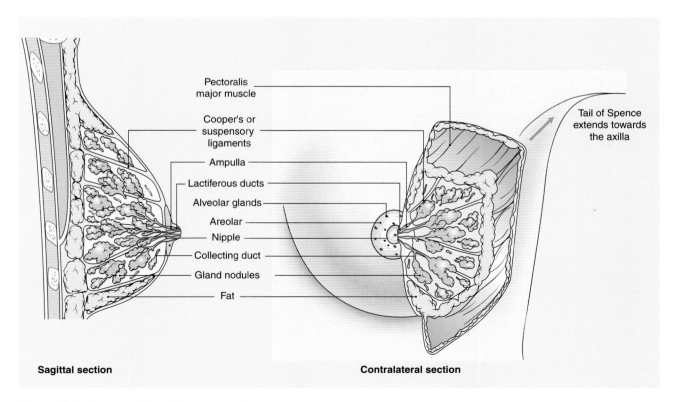

Pectoralis major muscle

Cooper's or suspensory ligaments

Ampulla

Lactiferous ducts

Alveolar glands

Areolar

Nipple

Collecting duct

Gland nodules

Fat

Tail of Spence extends towards the axilla

Sagittal section

Contralateral section

Figure 2.1 Cross section of the breast showing anatomy

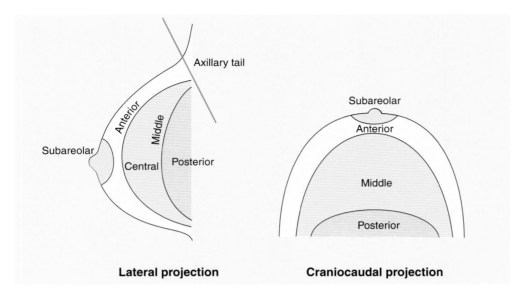

Lateral projection

Craniocaudal projection

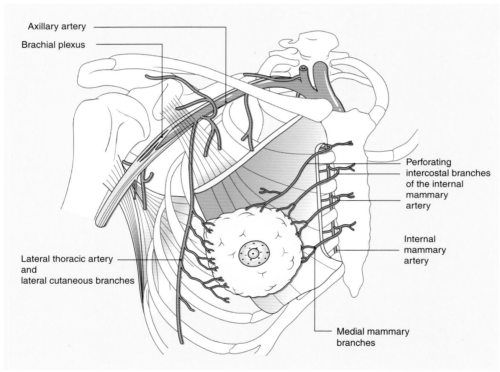

Figure 2.3 Vascular supply of the breast

from the nipple. Each lobe has one terminal excretory or collecting duct. The collecting ducts are 2 mm in diameter and converge into subareolar lactiferous sinuses or ducts that are 5–8 mm in diameter. Between five and ten major ducts drain to the outside through the nipple. The anatomical relationship of each lobe to its own unique terminal duct is important when evaluating multiple and single duct nipple discharge. Each lobe consists of 20–40 lobules, which each contain 10–100 alveoli. The alveoli are the secretory units of the breast.

Cooper's ligaments extend from the skin to the pectoralis major fascia. Shortening of Cooper's

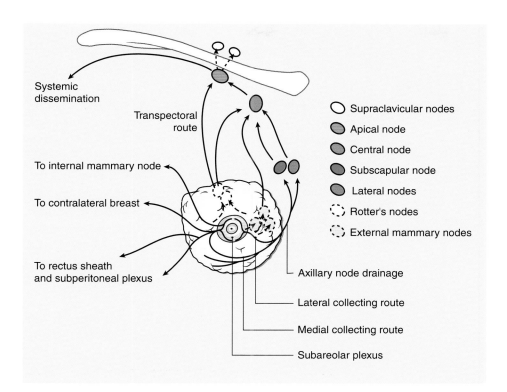

Figure 2.4 Lymphatic drainage of the breast.

Figure reproduced with permission from Pomrell LJ, Bland KI. Anatomy of the breast, axilla, chest wall and related metastatic sites. In Copeland EM, Bland KI, eds. *The Breast*. Philadelphia: WB Saunders, 1998:32

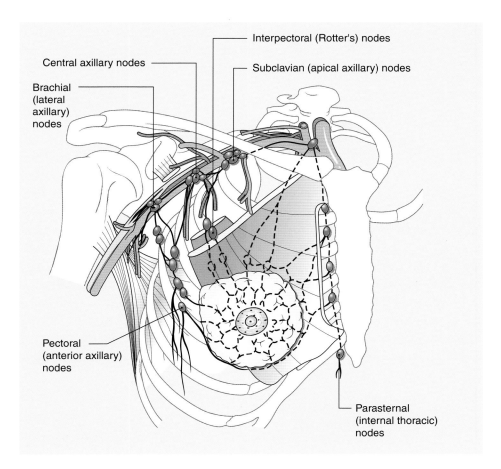

Figure 2.5 Anatomical lymphatic node groups of the breast

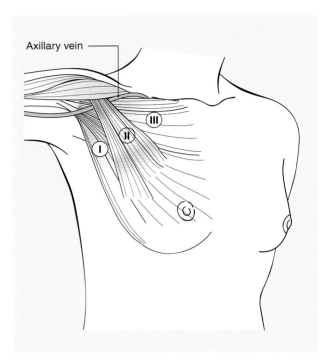
Axillary vein

Figure 2.6 Breast lymph nodes are divided into three anatomical levels. Level I is lateral to the pectoralis muscle. Level II is beneath the pectoralis minor muscle and Level III is medial to the pectoralis muscle. Level I and II lymph nodes are removed in the standard axillary dissection for breast cancer. The sentinel lymph node is usually in Level I. It is unusual for breast cancer to skip to higher levels of lymph nodes without involving lower levels

ligaments by tumor growth will result in skin retraction.

The nipple is located over the fourth intercostal space and contains sebaceous and apocrine sweat glands as well as nerve endings. The areola is the circular pigmented tissue around the nipple and contains the sebaceous glands of Montgomery, which are capable of secreting a milk-like substance. Morgagni's tubercles are elevations on the surface of the areola that are formed by the openings of the Montgomery gland duct.

Accessory breast tissue and nipples may occur along the breast line running from the axilla to the groin. Accessory breast tissue may be functional but it is usually rudimentary.

The vascular supply to the breast is from the internal mammary artery and lateral thoracic artery (Figure 2.3). The internal mammary artery primarily supplies the medial and central portion of the breast while the lateral thoracic artery supplies the upper outer quadrant.

Approximately 75% of the lymphatic drainage is to axillary nodes with most of the remaining 25% to internal mammary nodes and skin lymphatics (Figure 2.4). The axilla contains 30–60 lymph nodes which are divided into three anatomical levels: Level I nodes are lateral to the pectoralis minor muscle; Level II nodes are beneath the pectoralis minor muscle; and Level III nodes are medial to the pectoralis minor muscle. Interpectoral nodes (Rotter's nodes) are found between the pectoralis major and minor muscles (Figure 2.5). Lymphatic drainage proceeds sequentially from levels I to III and skip metastases from a lower to higher level are rare. Sentinel lymph node mapping for staging relies on orderly progression of lymph drainage from lower to higher nodal groups (I to III). Figure 2.6 illustrates axillary lymph node Levels I–III.

Internal mammary nodes are found in the intercostal spaces in the parasternal region. They are found close to the internal mammary vessels in the extrapleural fat. Lymphatic drainage proceeds from the internal mammary nodes to the intercostal nodes located posteriorly along the vertical column as well as subpectoral and subdiaphragmatic areas. Although lymphatic drainage usually proceeds in physiologic pathways, the tumor may spread through any pathway. Unusual drainage pathways may be explained by the tumor blocking the lymphatic routes, causing alternative routing and the direct spread of the tumor into various organs.

KEY POINTS: ANATOMY

1. The breast is composed of 15 to 20 lobes arranged in a radial fashion extending from the nipple
2. Each lobe of the breast has one unique terminal excretory duct which converges into subareolar lactiferous sinuses of which 5 to 10 drain outside through the nipple
3. The vascular supply of the breast is from the internal mammary artery and lateral thoracic artery
4. Approximately 75% of lymphatic drainage is to axillary nodes with the remaining 25% primarily to internal mammary nodes and skin lymphatics
5. Axillary lymphatic drainage proceeds from Level I to Level III and skip metastases are rare

SUGGESTED READING

Hall JA. *Breast Disorders: Obstetrics and Gynecology Principles and Practice*. Ling FW, Duff P, eds. New York: McGraw-Hill, 2001:938–54

Harris JR, Lippman ME, Morrow M, Hellman S, eds. *Diseases of the Breast*. Philadelphia: Lippincott-Raven, 1996

Hindle WH, ed. *Breast Care*. New York: Springer Verlag, 1999

CHAPTER 3

Physical examination

Breast examination is an important part of the routine clinical work-up. The patient should be examined unclothed in both the sitting and supine positions. The importance of breast self-examination can be emphasized at this time. Palpation should also include the axilla and supraclavicular areas. The entire breast and chest wall should be examined. The patient should be examined in the sitting position with the patient's arms raised over her head, hands pressing on the hips, and arms relaxed as the patient leans forward (Figure 3.1). The patient should then be examined

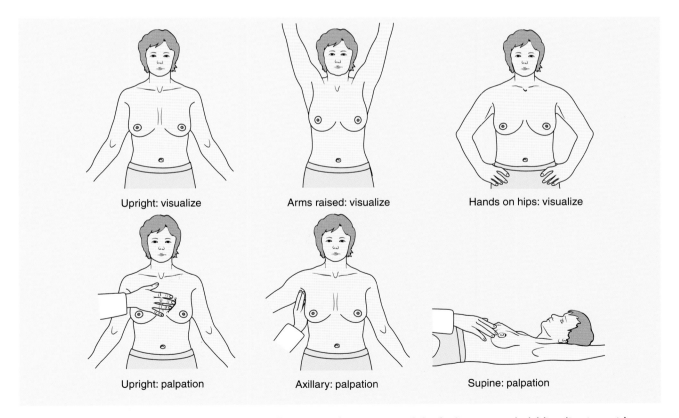

Upright: visualize   Arms raised: visualize   Hands on hips: visualize

Upright: palpation   Axillary: palpation   Supine: palpation

Figure 3.1 The patient is examined systematically in several positions and the findings recorded. Visualization with arms at sides and extended accentuates the effect of a tumor shortening the Cooper's ligaments with resulting flattening and concave appearance of the skin

on her back with her arms at her side as well as over her head. Clinical breast examination is best performed with circular motions using fingerpads (Figure 3.2). Tactile sensitivity may be improved when the breast is wet or with use of sonar gel.

Significant findings should be accurately noted in the medical record using standard drawings or templates (Figure 3.3). Vague statements or drawings of insignificant findings, such as dense areas, may be misinterpreted by others reviewing

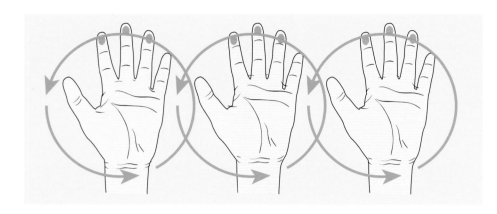

Figure 3.2 Clinical breast examination is best performed with circular motions using fingerpads. Tactile sensitivity may be improved when the breast is wet or with use of sonar gel

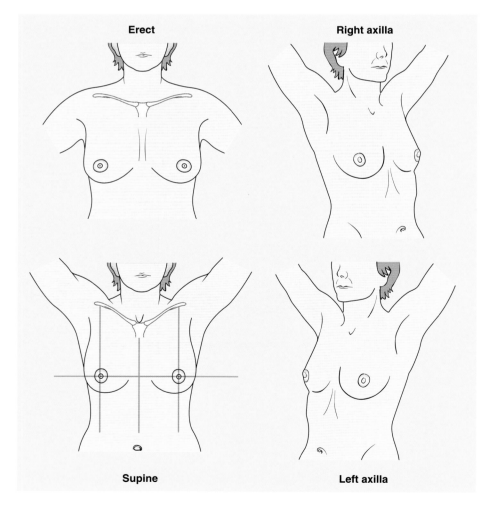

Erect

Right axilla

Supine

Left axilla

Figure 3.3 Standard drawings or templates are helpful to describe or locate physical findings. Only clinically significant findings should be recorded

the record and are damaging in a malpractice action. Use of the word 'mass' should be reserved for a structure that is clearly three-dimensional. Lumpy or asymmetrical areas should not be described as a mass. Drawings in the chart should not be used unless there are clinically significant findings. The location of a palpable mass is best described by using the clock face as a reference and the number of centimeters from the areolar edge (Figure 3.4). Charting must describe whether the patient's right or left breast is involved.

It is generally felt that a tumor must be 1 cm or larger to be reliably palpated. Dense, large, or lumpy breasts may hide tumors considerably larger than 1 cm. Growth rates predict that by the time an average breast cancer reaches a diameter of 1 cm, it has been present for 6–10 years. Breast cancers will rarely metastasize before reaching a diameter of 1 cm, a fact that validates the importance of mammographic screening.

Diagnostic steps should be promptly ordered and documented in the medical record. Physiologic changes, such as fibrocystic changes, should not be termed a 'disease'. Nipple discharge should be fully described, i.e. whether it is spontaneous or expressed, involving single or multiple ducts, unilateral or bilateral, and bloody or non-bloody (see Chapter 10). Chemical tests used to test stool specimens for blood may be helpful. Because each lobe has its own unique duct, the location of the origin of pathologic single duct nipple discharge can usually be determined by sequential pressure on the breast. The site of abnormality is nearly always subareolar or near the areolar edge. Locations distant in the periphery of the breast may be difficult to localize even with ductography. Although the cause of pathologic single duct nipple discharge is usually benign, malignancy must be excluded.

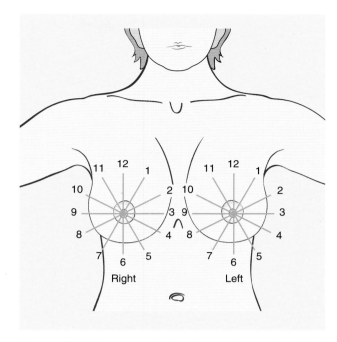

Figure 3.4 Location of the abnormality is described using the clock face and the number of centimeters from the areolar edge. It is important to record which breast is involved. Only significant findings should be charted

KEY POINTS: PHYSICAL EXAMINATION

1. Clinical breast examination is a necessary complement to screening mammography
2. Clinical breast examination is performed with the patient in both sitting and supine positions
3. Clinical breast examination is performed with circular motions using the fingerpads
4. Squeezing the nipple is painful and may stimulate clinically insignificant nipple secretion
5. The location of the abnormal duct producing pathologic nipple discharge can be found by noting which area of sequential palpation results in nipple discharge

SUGGESTED READING

Hall JA. *Breast Disorders: Obstetrics and Gynecology Principles and Practice*. Ling FW, Duff P, eds. New York: McGraw-Hill, 2001:938–54

Harris JR, Lippman ME, Marrow M, Heilman S, eds. *Diseases of the Breast*. Philadelphia: Lippincott-Raven, 1996

Hindle WH, ed. *Breast Care*. New York: Springer Verlag, 1999

CHAPTER 4

Breast imaging

MAMMOGRAPHY

There is widespread agreement regarding the benefit of mammographic screening every 1–2 years in women aged 50–69 years. Randomized trials have shown a 20–30% reduction in the risk of dying from breast cancer among screened women aged 50–69 years compared with unscreened women[1–3]. Recommendations for screening women aged 40–49 years are less obvious and less cost-effective, but remain beneficial. Breast cancer incidence is lower in the 40–49 year age group and the younger breast is more radiographically dense, making interpretation more difficult. The American College of Obstetricians and Gynecologists (ACOG) recommends screening women between 40–49 years of age every 1–2 years and

annually after age 50[4]. See Table 4.1 for screening guidelines. There is no agreement as to what age to discontinue screening protocols: as breast cancer incidence increases with age, it seems prudent to

Table 4.1 Recommended mammographic screening intervals

Screening should start at age 40 and be performed every 1–2 years and then annually after age 50
Safe age to increase screening interval has not been established
Earlier screening is recommended for women with first-degree relatives affected at an early age: • start screening 10 years earlier than the age of diagnosis of the affected relative • women with *BRCA 1* and *BRCA 2* mutations may want to start annual screening before age 40

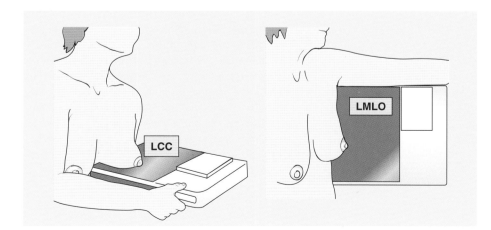

Figure 4.1 Standard screening mammograms include two views: craniocaudal (CC) and left mediolateral oblique (MLO), obtained by placing the film markers in the standard positions as shown. Diagnostic mammography investigates a specific problem or complaint by using special techniques such as different projections, spot compression, or magnification.

continue screening as long as the patient's health permits.

There are two types of mammogram imaging: screening and diagnostic. Screening is indicated for asymptomatic women and two standard views are taken (craniocaudal and mediolateral oblique; Figures 4.1–4.3). Diagnostic mammography is performed for a specific indication and includes specialized imaging views. Diagnostic mammography should be done for appropriate clinical indications and not deferred because of a patient's age.

Proper placement of the films for viewing is necessary (Figure 4.2) as mirror image comparison aids accuracy and detection of asymmetric areas. It is important to image the entire breast. Figure 4.3 illustrates quality assurance measures to ensure proper imaging position.

There is no evidence that current use of mammography increases the risk of breast cancer from radiation[5]. Mammography cannot be used to 'rule-out' cancer as around 10% of palpable tumors escape imaging detection and some non-palpable tumors fall below imaging capabilities. This reinforces the need for concordance in all parts of the diagnostic triad. The mammographic window[6] is the time in a life of a cancer when it can be discovered only with mammography (Figure 4.4). Only through screening mammography can tumors be discovered when they are

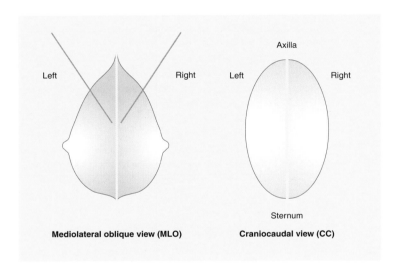

Figure 4.2 Proper positions for mammogram viewing. Mammogram films are viewed with similar projections as mirror images of both breasts. Comparison to previous studies is extremely valuable

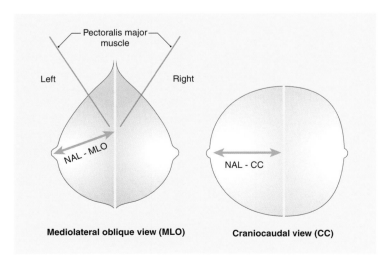

Figure 4.3 Proper breast positioning for imaging. It is important to image the entire breast. The pectoralis major muscle should be seen on the mediolateral oblique projection down to the level of the nipple axis line (NAL). Attempt should be made to see some pectoralis major muscle on the craniocaudal view to ensure imaging of the entire breast. The distance from the nipple to the back of the film on the craniocaudal view (NAL-CC) should be within I cm of the nipple axis line on the mediolateral oblique (NAL-MLO) view otherwise posterior breast tissue will not be imaged

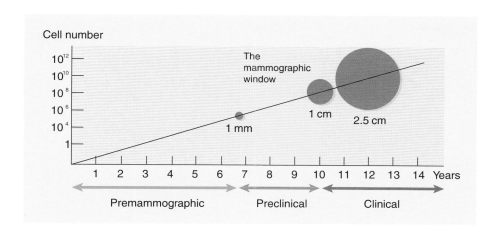

Figure 4.4 The mammographic window (as described by Wertheimer *et al.*[6]) is the period in the life of a breast cancer when it is discoverable only by mammographic imaging. Tumors are premammographic until they reach at least I mm and are not usually clinically palpable until at least I cm. Average growth rates predict it takes a breast cancer 6–10 years to reach I cm in diameter

Table 4.2 Breast imaging reporting and data system (BI-RADS) assessment categories

BI-RADS	
0	Need additional imaging evaluation
I	Negative study
2	Benign findings
3	Probable benign findings: short-term follow-up recommended
4	Suspicious abnormality: biopsy recommended
5	Highly suggestive of malignancy

For statistical review: BIRADS 0 ,4, 5 are considered 'abnormal'

Table 4.3 Desirable goals of mammogram audit data. Reproduced with permission from reference 8

PPVI (based on abnormal screening examination / BI-RADS 0, 4 ,5)	5–10%
PPV2 (when biopsy recommended / BI-RADS 4, 5)	25–40%
Tumors found – stage 0 or I	>50%
Tumors found – minimal cancer (< Imm or DCIS)	>30%
Node positivity	<25%
Cancer found/1000 asymptomatic women	2–10
Recall rate	<10%
Sensitivity (probability of detecting a cancer when a cancer exists)	TP / (TP+FN)
Specificity (number of mammographically normal cases in a population divided by all patients who did not have breast cancer in the population discovered within I year)	TP / (FP+TN)

PPV, Positive predictive value; TP, true positive; FN, false negative; FP, false positive; DCIS, ductal carcinoma *in situ*

small, early, and have minimal chance of metastases. A tumor 1 cm in diameter has probably existed for 6–10 years and carries a 40–50% chance of involvement of axillary nodes with metastatic disease.

Digital mammography and magnetic resonance imaging (MRI) hold promise to improve imaging capabilities. A clear and concise report from the radiologist is essential so there is no misunderstanding of the findings. Use of the American College of Radiology's *Breast Imaging Reporting and Data Systems*[7] (BI-RADS) assessment categories is advised (Table 4.2). Performance goals for mammogram centers are shown in Table 4.3. These centers are required to keep audit data in order to ensure quality imaging and follow-up.

The BI-RADS imaging lexicon evaluates each mammogram for the following characteristics:

(1) Mass

(2) Calcification

(3) Architectural distortion

(4) Special cases

(5) Associated findings

(6) Location of the lesion

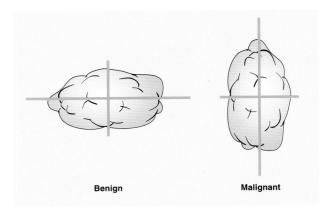

Benign   **Malignant**

Figure 4.5 Benign breast masses (cystic or solid) tend to orient themselves in a horizontal direction while malignant tumors usually orient vertically

Mass

A mass is a space-occupying lesion seen in two different projections. Lesions seen only on one projection are called a density. The description of a mass should include its location, shape, margins, and tissue density. Benign breast masses (cystic or solid) tend to orient themselves in a horizontal direction while malignant tumors usually orient vertically (Figure 4.5).

Calcifications

Benign calcifications are usually larger than calcifications associated with malignancy and are visible to the naked eye. Malignant calcifications are usually small, requiring a magnification lens to be seen. They can be grouped or clustered and pleomorphic or linear with or without fine branching. Benign calcifications may be found in the skin or vascular structures. They are usually homogeneous in shape and may be widely distributed throughout the breast. Benign calcification is less likely to be clustered than malignant calcification. Fibroadenoma may contain calcium which can be easily diagnosed with mammography due to its 'popcorn' appearance. Crescent-shaped calcium floating in a benign cyst can be seen on the straight lateral projection thus confirming that a mass is cystic. Serial mammography over several years or special views such as spot compression, different projections, or magnification views may be used to evaluate calcification.

Architectural distortion

Mammography may be used to evaluate normal breast architecture and asymmetry by comparing one breast to another. A neoplasm may not be visible but may create an asymmetric density requiring further investigation.

Special cases

A solitary dilated duct or inframammary lymph node may be visible. Lymph nodes are typically stable over time, located in the upper outer quadrant, and have a low density or 'notched-out' center.

Associated findings

Mammography can easily detect skin or nipple retraction, skin or trabecular thickening, skin lesions, or axillary adenopathy. These findings may be important as they may result from a breast abnormality or create misleading mammogram findings.

Location of the lesion

The exact location of the lesion should be noted using anatomic terms and the clock face as a reference (Figure 3.4). The report should clearly state which breast is being described. The location description includes right or left breast, clock face reference, and quadrant. The location may be central, subareolar, or axillary. The depth from the surface is either anterior, middle or posterior (Figure 2.2). The upper half of the breast may be described as superior and the lower inferior. Marking of the nipple is valuable to create a reference point. A diagnostic report is helpful to document positive findings (Figure 4.6).

Mammogram examples and clinical outcomes are shown in Figures 4.7–4.18. Abnormal areas are marked on the films.

BREAST DIAGNOSTIC REPORT

Name: _____   Date: _____

Age: _____   G _____   P _____   A _____   Referred by: _____

Reason for visit:

Mass: _____   MammoLesion: _____   Pain: _____   Nipple discharge: _____   Other: _____

Right/left history: _____

_____

Past breast history: _____

_____

Family history: _____

_____

BREAST ULTRASOUND   yes/no

Approximate location of abnormality

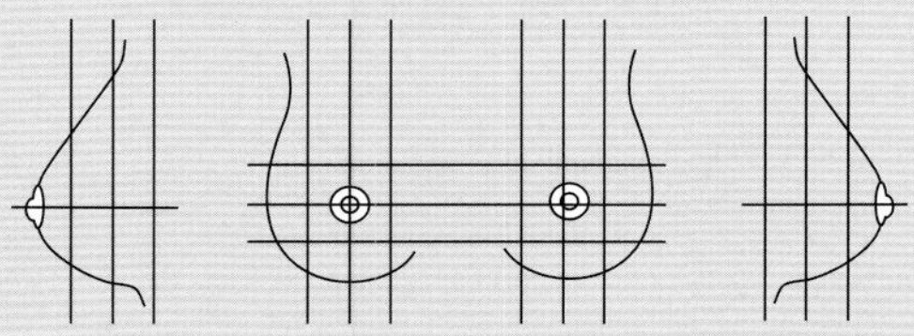

Right   Left

Findings: _____

Recommendations: _____

NEEDLE ASPIRATION yes/no

Solid / Cyst   Fluid: _____cc. Color: _____

Blood: yes / no   Resolution: yes / no

Cytology: yes / no

Cytology result: yes / no

Recommendation: _____

Approximate location of abnormality

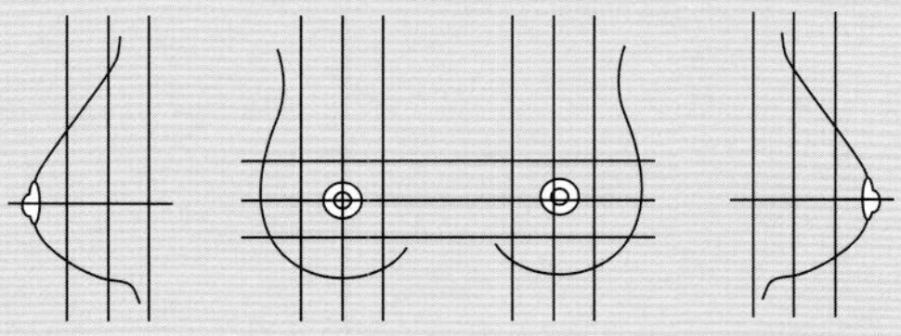

Right   Left

WOMEN'S HEALTH CENTER OF LOGANSPORT, 1025 MICHIGAN AVENUE, SUITE 115, LOGANSPORT, INDIANA 46947

TEL: 574/722-3566; FAX: 574/753-6113

Figure 4.6 Sample breast diagnostic report for recording results. Templates are beneficial to record the location of abnormalities. Only clinically important findings should be recorded. All findings and evaluation must be accurately recorded in the medical record

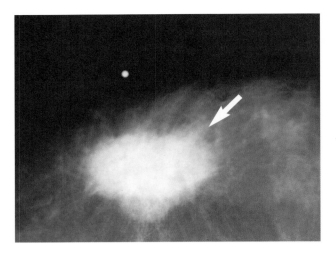

Figure 4.7 A 56-year-old presented with a 2 cm palpable mass in the right breast. Mammogram reveals a solid mass with irregular, speculated margins compatible with a BI-RADS 5 lesion. Biopsy confirmed infiltrating ductal carcinoma

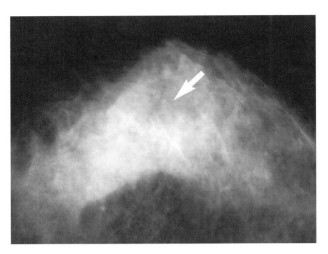

Figure 4.8 A 60-year-old whose screening mammogram revealed fine, granular, pleomorphic calcification suspicious for malignancy (BI-RADS 4). Wire localized biopsy revealed infiltrating ductal carcinoma of the left breast

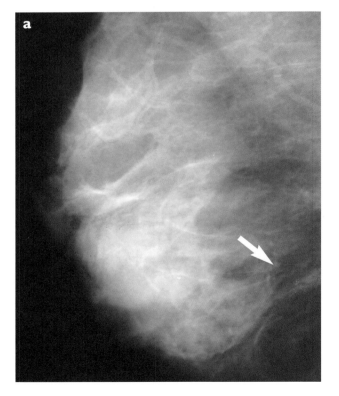

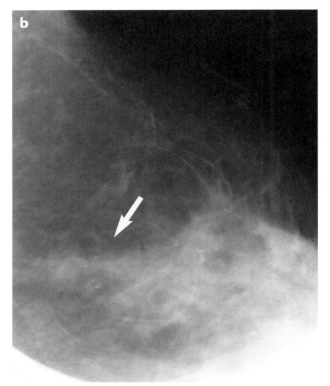

Figure 4.9 Screening mammogram of a 50-year-old woman. (a) Right mediolateral oblique view revealing an ill-defined area with microcalcifications that is poorly seen and could have been easily overlooked. (b) Spot compression magnification mediolateral oblique view showing a BI-RADS 4 area with small clustered pleomorphic calcifications. Stereotactic core-needle biopsy confirmed invasive ductal carcinoma

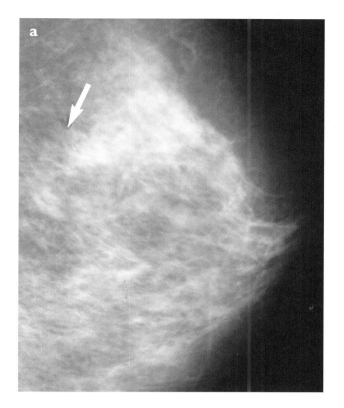

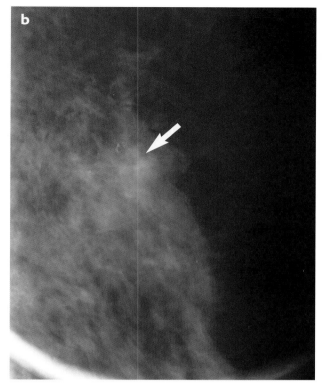

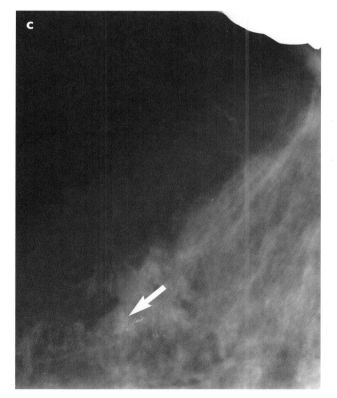

Figure 4.10 (a) Left mediolateral view from a screening mammogram of a 65-year-old woman. Suspicious lesions were noted with possible mass effect. (b) Mediolateral oblique and (c) magnification views confirm a clustered microcalcified lesion exhibiting pleomorphism and a possible mass. Biopsy was recommended and stereotactic core-needle biopsy confirmed a small invasive ductal carcinoma

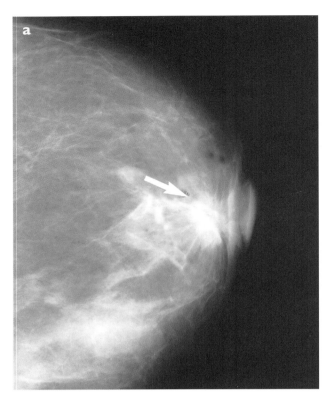
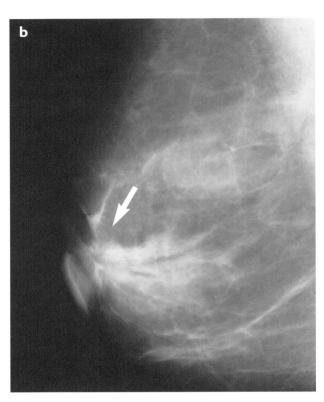

Figure 4.11 Screening mammogram of a 50-year-old reveals a solid spiculated mass immediately under the nipple/areola. There was no palpable or visible abnormality. Stereotactic core-needle biopsy revealed infiltrating ductal carcinoma. Tumor was discovered microscopically in multiple ducts under the nipple and on the surface of the areola. Modified radical mastectomy was required

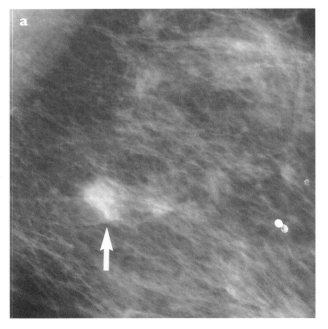
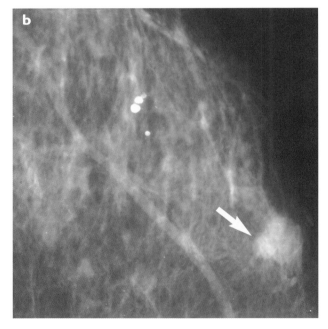

Figure 4.12 Screening mammogram of a 60-year-old with no palpable abnormality revealed a BI-RADS 4 mass with irregular margins in the mid-medial aspect of the left breast. Stereotactic core-needle biopsy revealed infiltrating ductal carcinoma

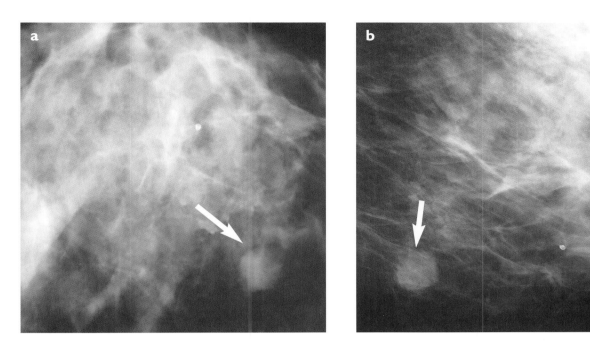

Figure 4.13 Screening mammogram of a 65-year-old revealed a mass in the 7 o'clock position of the left breast. The mass appeared solid with fairly smooth margins. Ultrasound failed to image a mass and biopsy was recommended. Stereotactic core-needle biopsy revealed a benign fibroadenoma

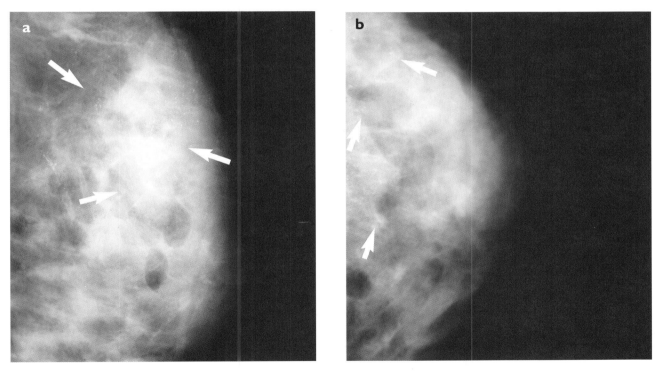

Figure 4.14 A 34-year-old woman, 3 months postpartum, presented with a bloody left nipple discharge. She was breastfeeding and there was no palpable mass. Mammogram revealed widespread suspicious BI-RADS 4, pleomorphic microcalcifications with linear and branching pattern. Biopsy revealed ductal carcinoma *in situ* with areas of micro-invasion. Left modified radical mastectomy was performed and approximately 70% of the breast was involved with ductal carcinoma *in situ* and rare areas of microinvasion. The axillary lymph nodes were negative

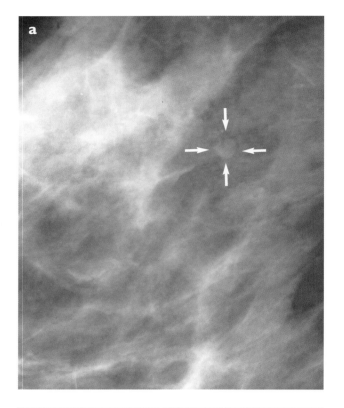

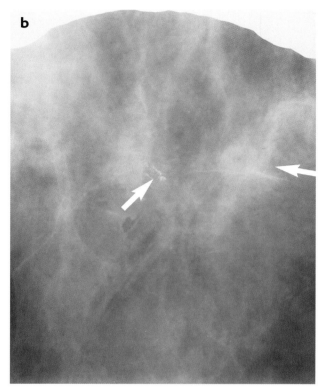

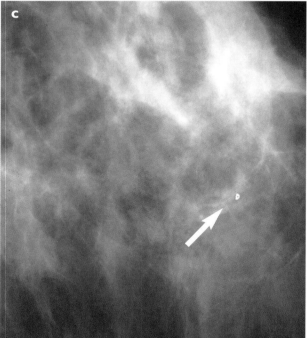

Figure 4.15 Screening mammogram of a 45-year-old woman revealed (a) a right breast suspicious micro-calcified area and an adjacent mass. (b) Magnification views confirmed a BI-RADS 4 clustered microcalcified area. The adjacent mass has smooth margins and a 'notched-out' low density center suspicious for a lymph node. Stereotactic core-needle biopsy was carried out and the microcalcified lesion was benign fibrocystic tissue and the mass was confirmed to be a lymph node. (c) Right mediolateral oblique view taken 1 year later confirmed removal of the microcalcified lesion and the lymph node. The clip placed at the time of biopsy to mark the area is seen

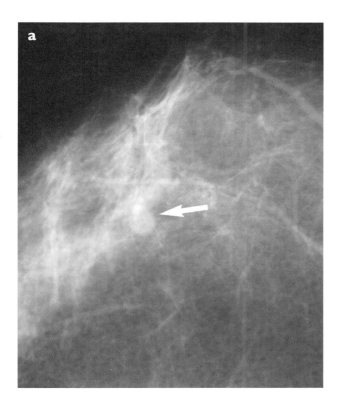

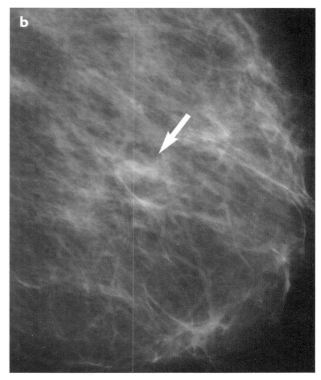

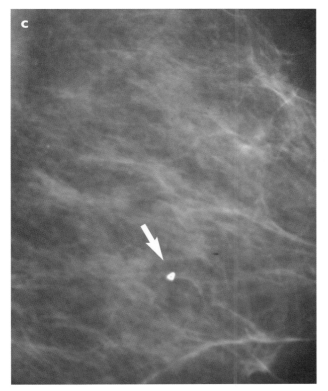

Figure 4.16 (a and b) Screening mammogram on a 42-year-old woman shows a 1 cm soft tissue mass in the mid-lateral left breast. The margins are smooth and the mass has a 'halo' appearance around the margin, suggestive of fibroadenoma. Ultrasound revealed an 8 mm solid mass corresponding to the mammogram mass. Stereotactic core-needle biopsy confirmed a benign fibroadenoma. (c) Mediolateral oblique post-biopsy film confirmed removal of the mass and a clip marking the location is seen

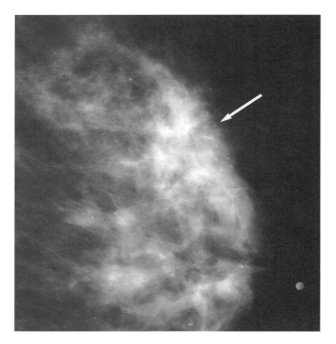 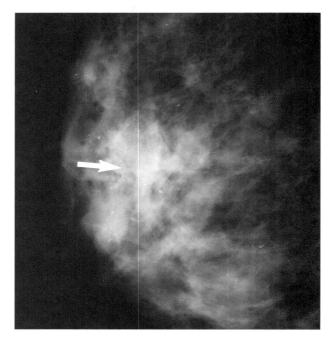

Figure 4.17 A 70-year-old female with a thick ridge along the mid-outer left breast. Mammography shows dense fibroglandular tissue which is confirmed to be fat necrosis on biopsy

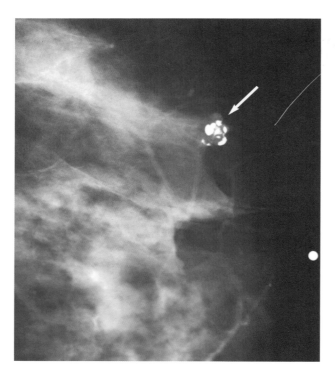

Figure 4.18 Screening mammogram (left craniocaudal view) reveals a classic 'popcorn' calcification associated with fibroadenoma

KEY POINTS: MAMMOGRAPHY

1. Proven to save lives in early detection of breast cancer
2. No significant radiation risk
3. Will discover 90% of breast cancers
4. Absence of radiographic signs of malignancy does not rule out breast cancer, especially with a palpable mass
5. Approximately 20–30% of nonpalpable mammogram abnormalities recommended for biopsy (BI-RADS 4, 5) are malignant

ULTRASOUND

Breast ultrasound is an adjunct to mammography and has limited value as a screening modality (Table 4.4). A dedicated real-time hand held transducer with at least a 7.5 MHz head is required for accuracy. The primary value of ultrasound is to investigate a target lesion discovered by a mammogram (Table 4.5). The following characteristics of a mass can be determined by ultrasound:

(1) Margins

(2) Background acoustic findings

(3) Internal echo patterns

(4) Echogenicity

(5) Compression effect on shape

(6) Compression effect on internal echoes.

Margins are described as either clear or irregular. Benign nodules usually have smooth, clear margins that are easily seen. Suspicious masses have margins that are difficult to see, lack clear definition, or are spiculated. Evaluation of the internal echo pattern and background acoustic pattern are used to determine if a mass is cystic or

Table 4.4 Breast ultrasound

Limited use in screening
Use as an adjunct to mammography to investigate a target lesion
Not needed for palpable mass as fine-needle aspiration will provide immediate feedback of whether the mass is cystic or solid
Cannot be used to evaluate microcalcifications seen on mammography
Radiographer must use dedicated equipment and have training in interpretation

Table 4.5 Breast ultrasound indications

Further investigation of a mammogram-discovered mass
Surveillance of abscess or postoperative seroma/hematoma
Guidance for needle aspiration or biopsy
Radiographic dense breast

Table 4.6 Criteria for ultrasound diagnosis of breast cyst (all must be satisfied)

Round or oval mass with well-circumscribed margins
Horizontal orientation that may flatten with compression
No internal echoes that suggest solid tissue
Enhanced through transmission with posterior acoustical enhancement of sound

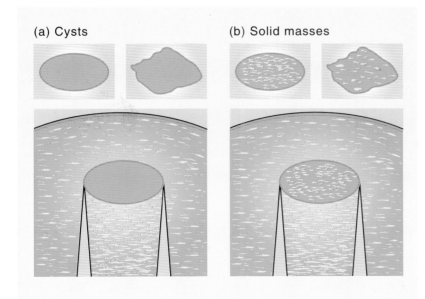

(a) Cysts   (b) Solid masses

Figure 4.19 Breast ultrasound illustrating differences between cystic and solid nodules. Cystic nodules have an anechoic center while solid masses demonstrate internal echoes. Cysts also have smooth margins, lateral shadowing, and are oriented transversely. Although solid masses may have benign features, it is not possible for ultrasound to differentiate between malignant and benign breast masses

Table 4.7 Ultrasound characteristics suggestive of malignant or benign solid masses. Data from reference 9

Malignant	Benign
Spiculation	Absent malignant findings
Angular margins	Intense hyperechogenicity
Marked hypoechogenicity	Ellipsoid shape
Shadowing	Gentle lobulations
Calcifications	Thin echogenic pseudocapsule
Duct extension	
Branch pattern	
Microlobulation	

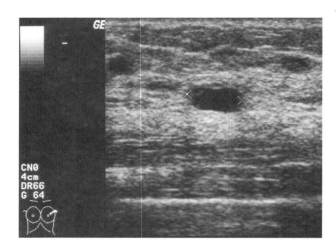

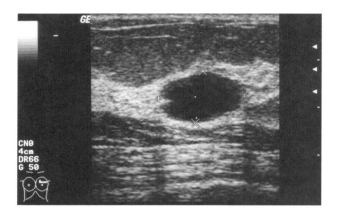

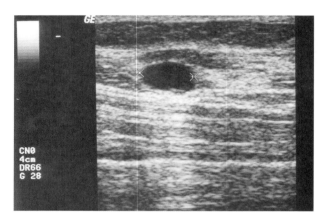

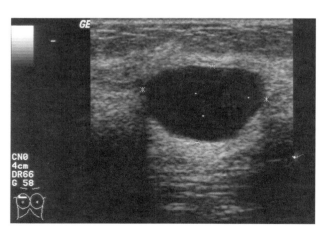

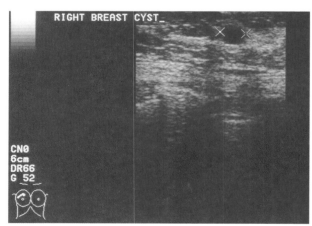

Figure 4.20 Breast ultrasound benign cysts. Ultrasound evaluation of non-palpable masses discovered by mammogram reveal benign cystic characteristics and can be safely observed

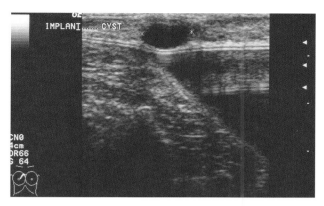

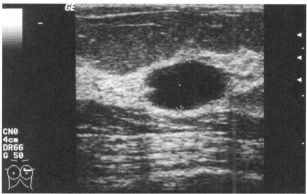

Figure 4.21 Breast cyst anterior to breast implant

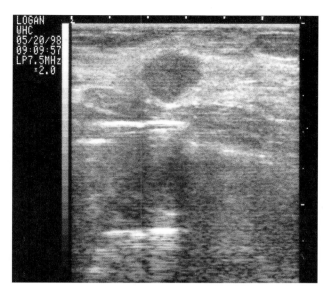

Figure 4.22 Ultrasound solid mass/breast carcinoma. Ultrasound evaluation of a non-palpable mammogram-discovered mass reveals solid characteristics. The internal architecture appears solid and the margins are irregular. The mass is oriented vertically and was confirmed to be malignant upon biopsy

solid. Compression will flatten a benign cyst and have minimal effect on a solid mass. Compression may make the internal appearance of a solid mass appear more dense and not alter a cystic mass.

A cystic mass may be observed while a solid mass will require tissue diagnosis. The rarity of cystic carcinoma makes ultrasound a valuable tool to investigate small non-palpable mammogram-discovered masses. Ultrasound cannot be used to evaluate areas of microcalcification. Palpable masses can be immediately needle-aspirated and do not require ultrasound investigation to determine if the mass is cystic or solid. Strict adherence to the criteria differentiating cystic from solid masses is essential (Table 4.6 and Figure 4.19). Current technology does not enable the use of ultrasound to determine if a solid mass is malignant or benign (Table 4.7)[8]. Ultrasound may also be used for guidance for needle aspiration or core biopsy procedures.

Examples of cystic masses are shown in Figures 4.20 and 4.21. Figure 4.22 illustrates the ultrasound appearance of a solid mass.

REFERENCES

1. US Preventative Services Task Force. *Guide to Preventative Services. Report of the US Preventative Services Task Force.* Baltimore: Williams and Wilkins, 1996

2. Fletcher FW, Black W, Harris R, *et al.* Report of the international workshop on screening for breast cancer. *J Natl Cancer Inst* 1993;85:1644–56

3. Sox HC. A tale of two consensus conferences: the controversy over breast cancer screening guidelines for women 40–50 years of age. *Sci Am Med Bull* 1997; 20(7)

4. ACOG Committee Opinion, The American College of Obstetricians and Gynecologists; 247:December 2000

5. Kopans DB, ed. *Breast Imaging.* Philadelphia: Lippincott-Raven, 1998

6. Wertheimer MD, Constanza ME, Dodson TF, *et al.* Increasing the effort toward breast cancer detection. *J Am Med Assoc* 1986;255:1311

7. American College of Radiology. *Breast Imaging Reporting and Data System (BI-RADS)*, 3rd edn. Reston, VA: American College of Radiology, 1998

8. Bassett LW, Hendrick RE, Bassford TL, *et al. Quality Determinants of Mammography. Clinical Practice Guideline no. 13*. Rockville, MD: Agency for Health Care Policy and Research, Public Health Service, US Department of Health and Human Services, October 1994; AHCPR publication no. 95-0632

9. Stavros AT, Thickman D, Rapp CL, *et al.* Solid breast nodules: use of sonography to distinguish between benign and malignant lesions. *Radiology* 1995;196: 123–34

KEY POINTS: BREAST ULTRASOUND

1. Must be performed with dedicated equipment/ has little use in screening
2. Adjunct to mammogram investigation of non-palpable mass
3. Used to differentiate cystic from solid masses
4. Used to guide needle aspiration or biopsy of non-palpable masses
5. Cannot reliably determine if a solid mass is malignant or benign

CHAPTER 5

Fine needle aspiration of the breast

Use of fine needle aspiration (FNA) will provide immediate knowledge of whether a palpable mass is cystic or solid. A cyst that contains non-bloody fluid, completely resolves with aspiration, and does not recur, is benign and does not need to be removed (Figure 5.1).

Cytology is not obtained on non-bloody fluid as it may produce misleading cytology findings.

Cyst fluid may be many different colors (Figure 5.2), however, the color is not important unless blood is present. Intracystic carcinoma occurs in only one in 1000 palpable cysts and the fluid is rarely cytologically diagnostic. Non-traumatic grossly bloody fluid from cyst aspiration is suspicious for carcinoma and requires a tissue diagnosis.

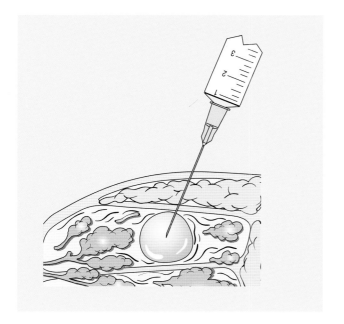 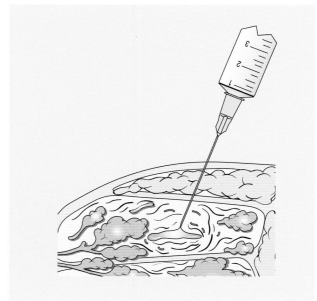

Figure 5.1 (a) Fine needle aspiration of breast cyst using 23-gauge needle and 10 cc syringe without anesthesia; (b) needle drainage of cyst

Fine needle aspiration of solid masses can make an accurate cytological diagnosis in at least 90% of tumors (Figure 5.3). It is also possible for the experienced clinician to differentiate between alternative types of masses according to the tactile sensations felt on entering the breast mass with the needle (Table 5.1). It is essential that the cytology sample contains an adequate volume of ductal cells. Inadequate specimens cannot be relied upon for diagnosis (Table 5.2)[1]. An accurate diagnosis also requires proper needle placement into the target lesion so that false-negative

Table 5.1 Tactile sensation felt on needle insertion into breast mass

Normal breast	Soft, no resistance
Fibrocystic changes	Intermittent, thick and soft
Cyst	Sudden loss of resistance with 'pop' upon entry
Fibroadenoma	Rubbery, similar to needle into eraser
Cancer	'Spitty', similar to needle into raw potato

Table 5.2 Fine needle aspiration cytology (FNAC). Reproduced with permission from reference 1

False-positive rate:
  less than 1% of cancers diagnosed (usually atypical fibro-adenomas or areas of prior radiation)
False-negative rate:
  less than 5% of cancers diagnosed (usually due to faulty technique)
Specimen inadequate for cytological diagnosis:
  too few cells; should be less than 5% of all aspirates
Atypical, borderline, or suspicious cells:
  need tissue through biopsy for definitive diagnosis. It is impossible to differentiate atypical cells, *in situ* carcinoma, or invasive disease
Conclusion:
  FNA with cytology will yield a specific diagnosis in 90% of palpable breast masses when there is an adequate cell sample

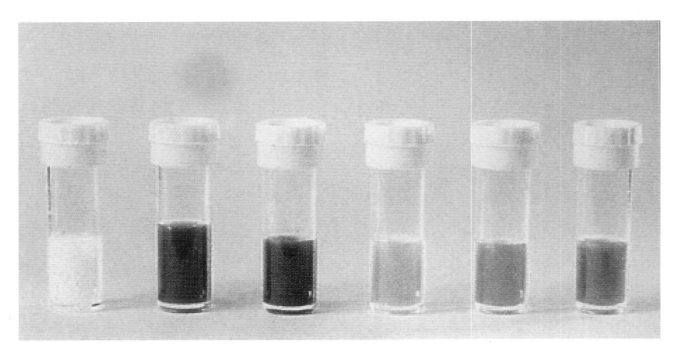

Figure 5.2 Colors of benign cyst fluid (courtesy of William Hindle, MD)

Table 5.3 Pitfalls to obtaining reliable results from fine needle aspiration

No true mass
Vague mass
Gross blood in syringe
Inadequate specimen: scant cells or acellular
Poor fixation of specimen
Gross fluid in syringe
Aspirated material clotted in syringe

information is not obtained (Table 5.3). The techniques involved in FNA are illustrated in Figures 5.3, 5.4 and 5.5.

Normal breast cytology

Four main cell types are found in the breast: epithelial, myoepithelial, adipose, and stromal (fibrous) (Table 5.4). One or more layers of

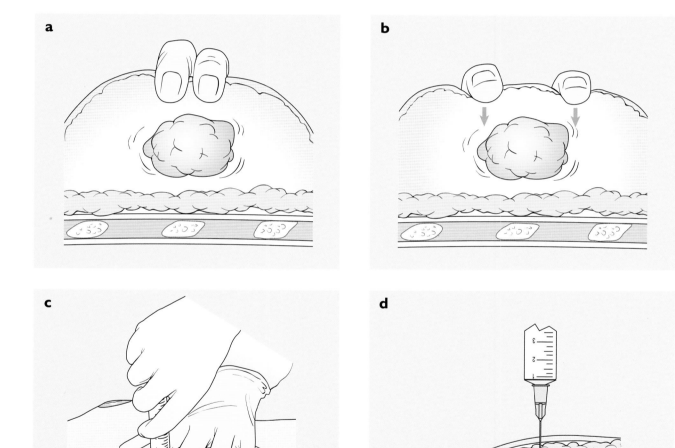

Figure 5.3 Fine needle aspiration of breast mass. (a) Breast mass is identified by palpation; (b) mass is stabilized and its location fixed between two fingers (fixing the mass over a rib is helpful); (c) stretching and tenting the skin between two fingers stabilizes the mass and reduces pain from the needle insertion; (d) needle tip is placed within the mass and tactile information from the resistance change on entering the mass confirms type of breast mass

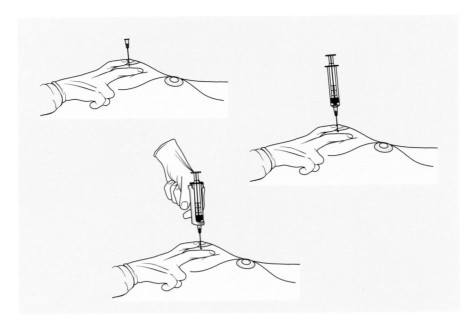

Figure 5.4 Fine needle aspiration of a small mass may be performed with a 23 gauge needle alone, needle and syringe, or needle and syringe attached to a piston grip device. In and out motion (bayonet thrusting) of the needle within the mass will result in cells coming into the needle

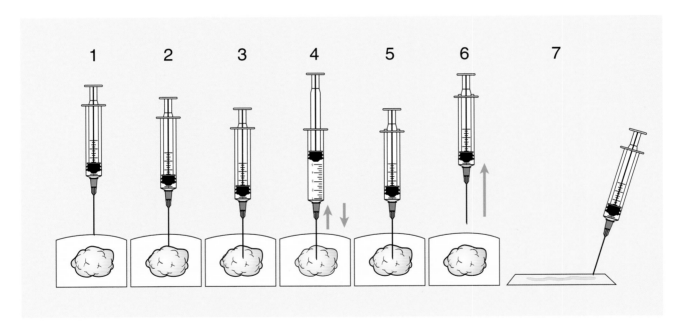

Figure 5.5 Fine needle aspiration of a solid mass for cytology (FNAC). Diagnostic mammogram (if indicated) should be obtained, if possible, before the needle aspiration to avoid hematoma formation, however the mammogram can be obtained immediately after the aspiration if it was non-traumatic. (1) Needle plunger is pulled back slightly before the aspiration in order to facilitate expression of the aspirated material. (2) The needle tip is placed within the mass. (3) An attempt should be made to place the tip of the needle into the middle of the mass. (4) Negative pressure (4–5 cc) is created by pulling back on the plunger and holding the position. The needle is thrust back and forth within the mass with short bayonet type movements for 10–20 passes. Care is taken to keep the needle within the mass and to avoid bleeding. The needle should be removed if traumatic blood appears within the needle hub and the available specimen prepared. Blood will compromise cytology interpretation. Repeat aspirations from another angle may be carried out in the event of traumatic bleeding. (5) Negative pressure is released while the needle is within the mass. The needle is withdrawn and pressure is applied at the aspiration site to reduce the chances of hematoma. (7) The tissue fluid containing cells will be within the needle and needle hub. The cells are expressed onto a slide or into cytology fluid and properly fixed

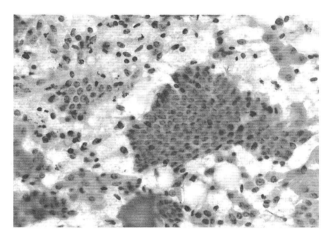

Figure 5.6 Benign cytology smear with normal cell patterns. Photograph courtesy of Kurt Hodges, MD

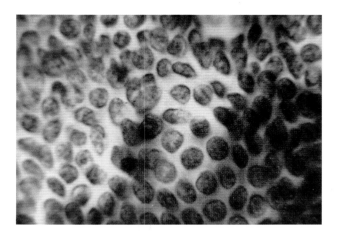

Figure 5.7 Fine needle aspiration cytology of fibroadenoma

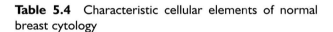

Table 5.4 Characteristic cellular elements of normal breast cytology

Small clumps of benign epithelial (ductal) cells
Stromal cells
Adipose cells
Widely distributed cellular elements

epithelial cells line the ducts and lobules and have secretory and absorptive roles. Myoepithelial cells are contractile and surround the ducts. Myoepithelial cells constrict and squeeze milk out of the lobules into major collecting ducts. They appear in cytology preparations as bipolar (elliptic-shaped) nuclei stripped of their cytoplasm. These naked or bare (without cytoplasm) nuclei are scattered singly throughout the smear and an abundant presence favors a benign process. Stromal cells, or fibroblasts, and adipose, or fat, cells compose most of the supporting structure of the breast ductal units. A benign cytology smear with normal cell patterns is shown in Figure 5.6.

Fibroadenoma

Fibroadenoma is a benign tumor of epithelial and connective tissue (Figure 5.7). Fine needle aspiration

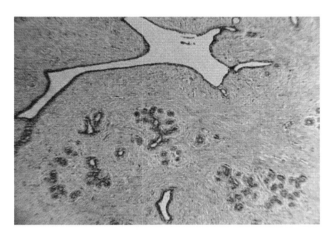

Figure 5.8 Histology of fibroadenoma

cytology of fibroadenoma shows the following characteristic features:

(1) Highly cellular smear

(2) Numerous sheets of monolayers of benign cohesive ductal cells

(3) Abundant bare naked bipolar nuclei representing myoepithelial cells

(4) Connective tissue stroma present

(5) Absence of adipose tissue.

Fibroadenomas are pseudoencapsulated and distinctly separate from the surrounding tissues

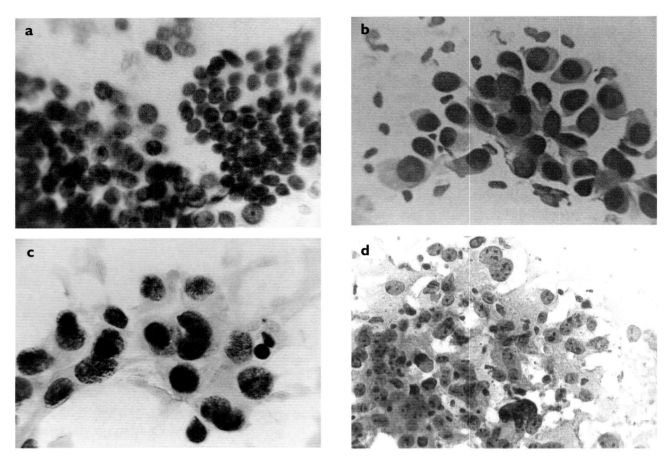

Figure 5.9 Fine needle aspiration cytology of invasive breast carcinoma. Figure 5.9d courtesy of Kurt Hodges, MD

(Figure 5.8). They are usually spherical or ovoid and have a microscopic appearance of epithelial and stromal components. The epithelial component consists of well-defined glandular duct spaces lined by cuboidal or columnar cells with uniform nuclei. Epithelial hyperplasia may be observed.

Invasive breast carcinoma

Adenocarcinoma is the most common malignancy of the breast and arises from epithelial cells (Figures 5.9 and 5.10). Characteristic cytology hallmarks of fine needle aspiration cytology of adenocarcinoma include:

(1) Abundant cellular elements

(2) Debris in the background giving the smear a 'dirty' appearance

(3) Loose attachment of the cancer cells to each other (dyshesion)

(4) Pleomorphism (variable size and shape) of the nuclei with hyperchromasia and prominent nucleoli

(5) Single cells with malignant features

(6) Red and white blood cells

(7) Occasional stroma

(8) Adipose tissue may be present.

Intracystic carcinoma

Intracystic carcinoma is rare and only found in approximately 1:1000 breast cysts. Cysts that contain non-traumatic bloody fluid, do not resolve with aspiration, or recur after two or more

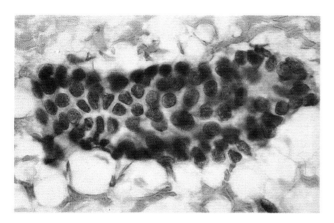

Figure 5.10 Fine needle aspiration cytology revealing malignant ductal epithelium with tubular carcinoma

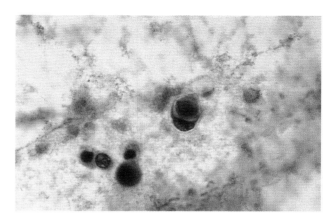

Figure 5.11 Fine needle aspiration cytology: intracystic carcinoma

aspirations should be evaluated with tissue biopsy to exclude malignancy. Cytology on non-bloody cyst fluid will usually not discover malignant cells even if a cancer is present. Confusing atypical cells may be seen from benign cysts and therefore cytology is best not obtained. Figure 5.11 shows malignant cells on aspirate from a rare intracystic carcinoma that contained non-traumatic bloody fluid.

REFERENCE

1. Hindle WH, ed. *Breast Care*. New York: Springer Verlag, 1999

KEY POINTS: FINE NEEDLE ASPIRATION OF THE BREAST

1. Fine needle aspiration (FNA) is an important part of the diagnostic triad along with physical examination and mammography
2. FNA can immediately diagnose a breast cyst without the need for ultrasound, mammography, or referral
3. FNA is an office procedure that requires no anesthesia and is virtually painless
4. FNA with cytology (FNAC) of a solid mass has a low false-negative rate and rare false-positive rate when an adequate ductal cell sample is obtained
5. FNAC is non-diagnostic without an adequate ductal cell sample

CHAPTER 6

Breast biopsy techniques

While complete removal of an abnormal breast lesion by excisional biopsy remains the gold standard in breast disease diagnosis, an array of less invasive techniques are available to determine the nature of a palpable or imaged detected breast abnormality. The widespread use of screening mammography and breast ultrasound has resulted in detection of non-palpable lesions amenable to fine needle, core needle and large bore excisional breast biopsy. All of these techniques have reduced the incidence and need for open biopsy for suspicious breast lesions.

NON-PALPABLE BREAST LESIONS

Extensive use of screening mammography and breast ultrasound has dictated the need for less invasive breast tissue sampling techniques. Image-guided (mammography or ultrasound) core needle biopsy has become standard in obtaining a diagnosis when these lesions are detected. As most image-detected lesions are benign, these image-guided techniques have markedly reduced the need for open biopsy.

STEREOTACTIC CORE NEEDLE BIOPSY

Stereotactic core needle biopsies (SCNB) are done with X-ray imaging of mammographically detected, non-palpable breast lesions. Lesion localization is done by triangulation on a unit dedicated to SCNB. Breast abnormalities that are appropriate for SCNB are noted in Table 6.1. Contraindications to SCNB are noted in Table 6.2.

Briefly, the technique of SCNB involves multiple core biopsies taken with an 11-gauge needle utilizing a spring-loaded biopsy gun. Multiple core

Table 6.1 Abnormalities that are candidates for stereotactically guided core needle breast biopsy. Reproduced with permission from reference 1

A solid, non-palpable mass associated with:
    Irregular shape
    Spiculated or ill-defined margins
    Microlobulations
    Suspicious calcifications
    Associated findings such as:
        Focal skin thickening
        Focal solitary dilated duct

Microcalcifications with the following features:
    Morphology – varying size or shape (pleomorphic), fine linear, branching, or granular
    Distribution – clustered (grouped), linear, or regional

An area of suspicious architectural distortion in a known prior biopsy site that demonstrates a suspicious interval change since a prior mammogram

Asymmetry associated with suspicious calcifications, architectural distortion, a non-cystic mass, a solitary dilated duct, or focal skin thickening

Solid, circumscribed mass that is dominant (usually larger than 1 cm) or shows interval growth since a prior mammogram

Table 6.2 Contraindications to stereotactically guided core needle biopsy. Reproduced with permission from reference 1

I. Lesions in the benign or probably benign category, such as:

Masses that:
    Are circumscribed, of low density, and smaller than 1 cm unless changed since the prior mammogram
    Contain intralesional fat of a density that is pathognomic for a lymph node, oil cyst, or hamartoma
    Are multiple, noncalcified, and circumscribed

Microcalcifications that are:
    Tiny, round or oval, uniform and in a localized cluster
    In a discrete cluster (or clusters) suggestive of milk of calcium, secretory disease, or sclerosing adenosis

II. Unequivocal, palpable masses

samples are taken, usually completely removing the image detected non-palpable lesion. Histopathology of these multiple core biopsies is highly accurate.

ULTRASOUND-GUIDED CORE NEEDLE BIOPSY

Non-palpable, suspicious breast abnormalities detected by ultrasound or visualized better than mammography on ultrasound are readily sampled by ultrasound-guided core needle biopsy. Real-time imaging of lesion sampling is utilized for documentation. Core samples recovered are handled identically to SCNB tissue cores.

NEEDLE (WIRE) LOCALIZATION OPEN BREAST BIOPSY

Some image detected non-palpable breast lesions are not amenable to SCNB. Lesions very close to the chest wall or areola may be inaccessible or too close to the chest wall to warrant safe SCNB. Prior to open biopsy excision, the non-palpable image detected lesion is localized by percutaneous placement of a barb-tipped localizing wire. Complete excision is confirmed by specimen mammography (Figure 6.1).

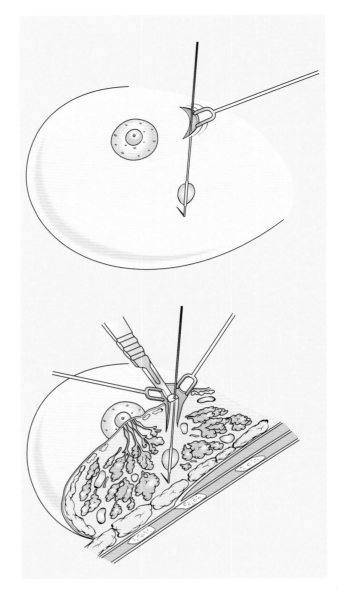

Figure 6.1 Needle-localized breast biopsy. The mammographic abnormality is localized immediately before operation. The relation between the wire, the skin entry site, and the lesion is noted by the surgeon. The skin incision is placed over the expected location of the mammographic abnormality. The dissection is accomplished with the wire as a guide. The tissue around the wire is removed en bloc with the wire and sent for specimen mammography. Reproduced with permission from Smith BL, Souba WW. Breast procedures. In *Scientific American Surgery*. NY: Scientific American, 1997

Table 6.3 Indications for open surgical biopsy. Reproduced with permission from reference 2

Bloody cyst fluid from aspiration

Failure of the mass to disappear after aspiration

Recurrence of a cyst after one or two aspirations

Non-palpable solid mass not diagnosed as fibroadenoma on core biopsy

Bloody nipple discharge

Nipple ulceration or persistent crusting

Skin edema or erythema suspicious for inflammatory breast carcinoma

OPEN BREAST BIOPSY

Occasionally, breast lesions present that are not appropriate for minimally invasive diagnostic needle or core needle biopsy (see Table 6.3). An open, excisional breast biopsy is designed to remove the abnormal lesion with some margin of normal breast tissue surrounding it (Figure 6.2). Open breast biopsy may be performed in an ambulatory setting under local anesthetic or in a surgical suite under general anesthesia depending on patient preference and lesion location. Placement of the open biopsy skin incision is strategic for an excellent cosmetic result (Figure 6.3). Additionally, should a malignant diagnosis be

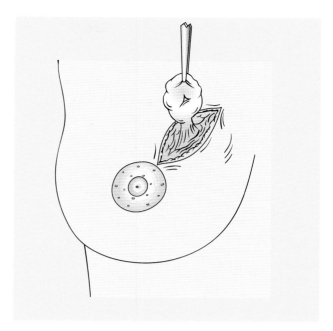

Figure 6.2 An excisional biopsy is intended to completely remove the abnormal lesion with a margin of surrounding normal breast tissue. Figure reproduced with permission from Strömbeck JO, Rosato FE, eds. *Surgery of the Breast: Diagnosis and Treatment of Breast Diseases.* Stuttgart, New York: Thieme, 1986

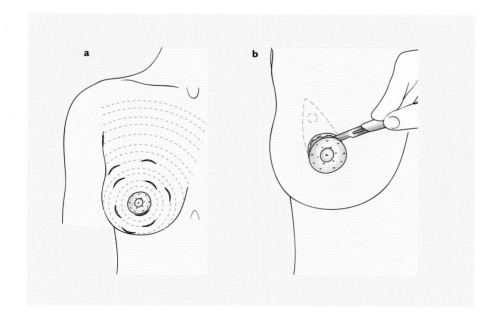

Figure 6.3 Recommended locations of incisions for performing breast biopsy. Cosmetically acceptable scars result from incisions that (a) follow the contour of Langer's lines, or (b) those placed around the areolar. Figure reproduced with permission from Bland KI, Copeland EM, eds. *The Breast: Comprehensive Management of Benign and Malignant Diseases,* 2nd edn. Philadelphia: WB Saunders, 1998

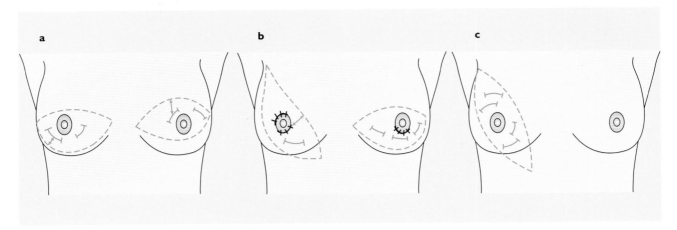

Figure 6.4 Incisions for breast biopsy are placed within the boundaries of skin flaps to be elevated if subsequent mastectomy is to be performed. (a) Transverse mastectomy incisions. Margins of the mastectomy incision are developed 1 to 2 cm from the margins of the curvilinear breast biopsy. (b and c) Oblique mastectomy incisions may be necessary for peripherally placed breast biopsy incisions. Figure reproduced with permission from Smith BL, Souba WW. Breast procedures. In *Scientific American Surgery*. NY: Scientific American, 1997

rendered on open biopsy, incision placement is strategic if subsequent mastectomy is deemed unnecessary (Figure 6.4).

Open breast biopsy techniques utilize standard sterile techniques, meticulous hemostasis and a cosmetic subcuticular skin closure. Lesion histopathology is critical with specimen margins usually oriented by the surgeon for the pathologist.

REFERENCES

1. Bassett L, Winchester DP, Caplan RB, *et al*. Stereotactic core-needle biopsy of the breast: A report of the Joint Task Force of the American College of Radiology, American College of Surgeons, and College of American Pathologists. *CA Cancer J Clin* 1997;47:171–90

2. Dolan JR, Wierda A. Breast biopsy: indications and techniques. *Operat Tech Gynecol Surg* 2000;5:128–37

3. Smith BL, Souba WW. Breast procedures. In *Scientific American Surgery*. NY: Scientific American, 1997

KEY POINTS: BREAST BIOPSY TECHNIQUES

1. Complete surgical excision of a dominant mass remains the cornerstone of breast disease diagnosis
2. A palpable breast mass may be surgically excised (open biopsy), sampled by fine needle aspiration (see Chapter 5), or core needle biopsied for diagnosis
3. Non-palpable (imaging detected) breast lesions may be biopsied by fine needle, core needle or large core needle utilizing imaging-guided techniques (stereotactic core needle biopsy)
4. Duct excision is performed for intraductal papillomas

CHAPTER 7

The pathology of breast disease

BREAST DEVELOPMENT

The female breast undergoes dramatic changes in size, shape and function during growth, puberty, pregnancy, lactation, and postmenopausal regression. Lobular formation occurs at puberty, but the completion of breast development and cellular differentiation occurs only at the end of a full-term pregnancy. With pregnancy, the mammary parenchyma reaches its final stages of development with secretory lobules. It is postulated that the induction of cellular differentiation of the breast by pregnancy is partially responsible for the inhibition of carcinogenic initiation.

Each breast is composed of 15–20 segmented units. Large ducts progressively branch into sub-segmental ducts that end as terminal ductal-lobular units (TDLU) (Figure 7.1)

Histologically, mammary epithelium is ecto-dermally derived and is composed of an inner epithelial cell layer and an outer myeoepithelial layer that separates the epithelial cells from the basement membrane. The epithelial cells of the TDLU are hormonally responsive and undergo secretory change for lactation.

FIBROCYSTIC CONDITIONS

The term fibrocystic condition is applied to a broad spectrum of morphological changes in the female breast ranging from completely benign (see Table 7.1) to those associated with an increased risk of carcinoma. Clinically, fibrocystic condition can produce palpable abnormalities in the breast tissue. Sixty to ninety percent of patients undergoing

Table 7.1 Benign breast conditions

Major ducts
Galactorrhea
Galactocele
Duct ectasia
Papilloma
Terminal ductal lobular unit
Fibrocystic conditions
cyst formation
Sclerosing adenosis
sclerosis of stroma
epithelial hyperplasia
Fibroadenoma
Other
Infection
Trauma
hematoma
fat necrosis

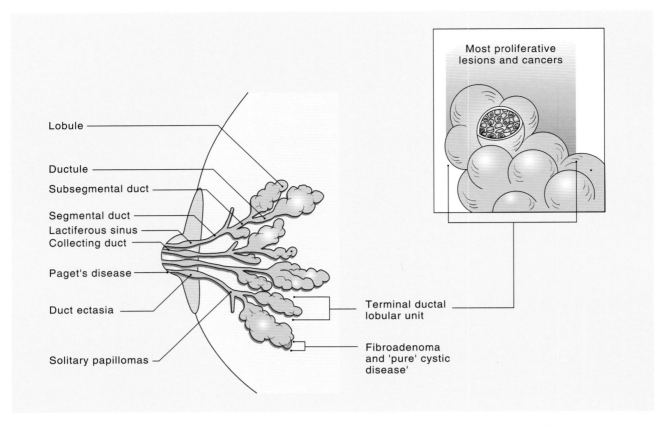

Figure 7.1 Correlation between anatomic structures and pathologic processes in the breast. Figure adapted with permission from Isaacs JH, ed. *Textbook of Breast Disease*. St Louis, MO: Mosby-Year Book, Inc., 1992

routine breast examination are considered to have fibrocystic condition (Figure 7.2), which runs through the morphologic spectrum from cysts, through fibrostroma, admixed stromal, and epithelial proliferation. Pathologists usually describe three dominant patterns in fibrocystic condition:

(1)   Cyst formation and fibrosis

(2)   Epithelial hyperplasia (ductal or lobular)

(3)   Sclerosing adenosis

The histologic variant most consistently associated with subsequent risk of carcinoma is epithelial hyperplasia. The progression from normal duct morphology through mild and atypical hyperplasia to carcinoma *in situ* is thought to precede invasive carcinoma (see Figure 7.3).

Table 7.2 depicts benign histology and relative risk of malignant potential.

BENIGN TUMORS

Several relatively common benign tumors are appropriate to mention. Fibroadenoma is the most common benign tumor of the female breast. It is composed of both fibrous and glandular tissue. The fibroadenoma grows as a well circumscribed, freely mobile breast mass. Most are between two and four centimeters in diameter when surgically removed but they can reach large sizes.

Phyllodes tumors arise from intralobular stroma and may be benign or frankly malignant. Clinical behavior is variable. Intraductal papilloma presents as a neoplastic papillary growth within a major duct. Serous or bloody nipple discharge is a common symptom. Treatment is complete excision of the involved duct.

CARCINOMA

Non-invasive intraductal (*in situ*) carcinoma represents malignant cells lacking the capacity to invade the basement membrane (Figure 7.4). They can, however, spread throughout the ductal system (see Table 7.3, Figure 7.5). Histologically, ductal carcinoma *in situ* (DCIS) is divided into five subtypes: comedocarcinoma, solid, cribiform,

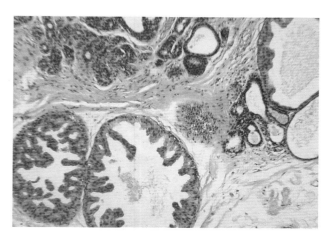

Figure 7.2 Fibrocystic condition of the breast

Table 7.2 Benign breast histology and relative risk of malignant potential

No increased risk	Slightly increased risk (1.5–2x)	Moderately increased risk (5x)	Markedly increased risk (10x)
Adenosis	Hyperplasia (moderate or florid, solid or papillary)	Atypical hyperplasia (ductal or lobular)	Carcinoma *in situ*
Apocrine metaplasia	Papillomatosis		Atypical hyperplasia with family history of breast cancer
Cysts			
Duct ectasia			
Fibroadenoma			
Fibrosis			
Hyperplasia, mild			
Mastitis			
Squamous metaplasia			

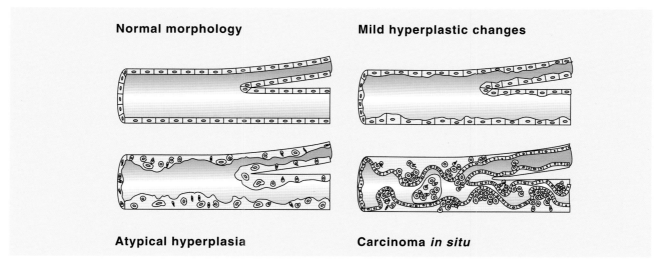

Figure 7.3 Schematic representation of the breast duct lining showing the progression from normal morphology, to mild hyperplastic changes, atypical hyperplasia and carcinoma *in situ*. Figure reproduced with permission from O'Grady LF, Lindfors KK, Howell LP, Rippon MB, eds. *A Practical Approach to Breast Disease*. Boston: Little, Brown, and Co., 1995

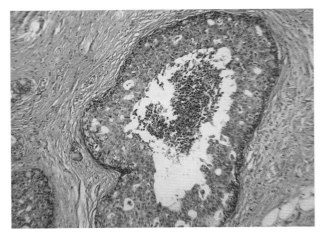

Figure 7.4 Ductal carcinoma *in situ* (DCIS) of the breast

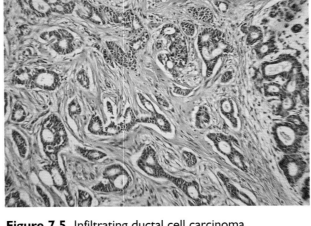

Figure 7.5 Infiltrating ductal cell carcinoma

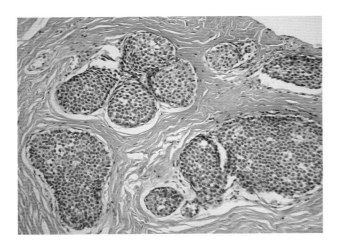

Figure 7.6 Lobular carcinoma *in situ*

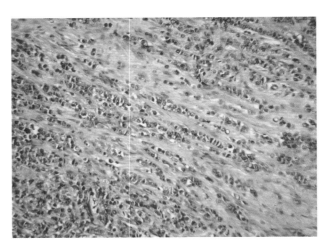

Figure 7.7 Infiltrating lobular carcinoma

papillary and micropapillary. Comedocarcinoma is characterized by rapidly proliferating malignant cells and aggressive treatment is warranted.

Lobular carcinoma *in situ* (LCIS) is manifested by histologic proliferation of well differentiated tumor cells contained in the terminal ducts (Figure 7.6). LCIS is considered a future marker of invasive breast cancer as 30% of LCIS will manifest itself later as invasive carcinoma, sometimes many years later.

Invasive duct cell carcinoma is characterized histologically by cords and solid nests of malignant cells which have broken through the basement membrane (see Figure 7.5). Clinically, invasive ductal carcinomas are characterized by cell type, size, grade, lymph node metastasis and a series of prognostic studies including hormone receptors and oncogene overexpression (see Table 7.3).

Invasive lobular carcinoma tend to be multicentric within the same breast. Often, the tumor is poorly circumscribed and, histologically, is characterized by strands of infiltrating tumor cells loosely arranged throughout the fibrous breast matrix. Invasive lobular carcinoma is characterized similarly to invasive duct cell carcinoma (Figure 7.7).

Table 7.3 Malignant breast conditions

Ductal cell carcinoma
Invasive (infiltrating) duct cell
Mucinous (colloid)
Tubular
Papillary
Medullary

Lobular carcinoma
Invasive (infiltrating) carcinoma

Rare forms of breast cancer
Adenoid cystic carcinoma
Secretory carcinoma
Stromal tumors
Phyllodes (cystosarcoma phyllodes)
Sarcoma
Metastatic tumor

SUGGESTED READING

National Comprehensive Cancer Network. Practice guidelines for breast cancer. *Oncology* 2000;14:33–49

KEY POINTS: PATHOLOGY OF BREAST DISEASE

1. Morphologic cellular changes of certain benign breast conditions are thought to proliferate resulting in the eventual formation of malignant breast cells (see Table 7.2)
2. Benign pathology of the breast may arise from major ducts or the terminal duct lobular units (TDLU) see Table 7.1 and Figure 7.1
3. Malignant diseases of the breast arise almost exclusively from the TDLU (see Table 7.3)

CHAPTER 8

Malignant breast disease risk factors

The presence or absence of risk factors should not alter the evaluation of a breast complaint (Table 8.1)[1]. The majority of women who develop breast cancer have no family history and less than 30% have any risk factor other than age or gender. Only 1% of breast cancers occur in men. The risk of breast cancer increases with age and 85% occur in women over 49 years. The commonly quoted statement that one in eight women will develop breast cancer can be misleading: this does not mean that one in eight women will have breast cancer at a specific point in time. What is meant is that for all women born in 1990 who live to be 95 years old, one in eight will develop breast cancer sometime during her lifetime. Two percent of women will develop breast cancer by age 50 and 5% by age 65.

The presence or absence of risk factors should not detract from the fact that all women are at risk for breast cancer. All breast complaints should be fully evaluated without any prejudice due to risk factors. Hereditary predisposition is a factor in only 5–7% of breast cancer cases.

BRCA 1 AND BRCA 2

A genetic predisposition to breast cancer has been recognized in some families. Between 5 and 7% of breast cancers are thought to result from mutations of tumor suppressor genes *BRCA 1* and

Table 8.1 Factors that increase the relative risk (RR) for breast cancer in women. Reproduced with permission from reference 1

RR	Factor
RR >4.0	Inherited genetic mutations for breast cancer
	Two or more first-degree relatives with breast cancer diagnosed at an early age
	Personal history of breast cancer
	Age (65+ vs. <65 years, although risk increases across all ages until age 80)
RR 2.1–4.0	One first-degree relative with breast cancer
	Nodular densities on mammogram (>75% of breast volume)
	Atypical hyperplasia
	High-dose ionizing radiation to the chest
	Ovaries not surgically removed < age 40
RR 1.1–2.0	High socioeconomic status
	Urban residence
	Northern US residence
Reproductive factors	Early menarche (<12 years)
	Late menopause (≥55 years)
	No full-term pregnancies (for breast cancer diagnosed at age 40+ years)
	Late age at first full-term pregnancy (≥30 years)
	Never breast-fed
Other factors that affect circulating hormones or genetic susceptibility	Postmenopausal obesity
	Alcohol consumption
	Recent hormone replacement therapy
	Recent oral contraceptive use
	Tall
	Personal history of cancer of endometrium, ovary, or colon
	Jewish heritage

Table 8.2 Effect of proliferative breast disease and family history (FH; first degree relative) on relative risk (RR) of breast cancer. Reproduced with permission from reference 2

	Proliferative disease no atypia		Atypical hyperplasia	
	No FH	FH	No FH	FH
Nurses' Health Study RR	1.3	4.5	3.7	7.3
Breast Cancer Detection Demonstration Project RR	1.7	2.6	4.2	22

BRCA 2. BRCA 1 is located on chromosome 17 and BRCA 2 on chromosome 13. Both are tumor suppressor genes where a mutation will increase the risk of cancer. The BRCA 1 and BRCA 2 frequency in the general population is low, occurring in one in 800 individuals. However, 50 to 80% of women who inherit either a BRCA 1 or BRCA 2 mutation will develop breast cancer by age 70. The risk of ovarian cancer is also increased for women who have inherited these mutations and is estimated to be 15–20% by age 70. BRCA 1 confers a higher ovarian risk than BRCA 2. Multiple mutations and variable penetration of the mutations make it difficult to recommend clinical use of these genetic tests. Approximately 600 BRCA 1 and 500 BRCA 2 mutations have been found, of which 70–80% are thought to produce disease. Unfortunately the exact biological function of BRCA 1 and BRCA 2 is still unknown. The importance of a positive test result in the absence of a strong family history is unclear. BRCA 2 is responsible for a higher risk of breast cancer in men.

On learning they carry one of these mutations patients will have to decide either to be followed with close surveillance, elect for prophylactic removal of the breasts or ovaries, or accept a trial of chemoprevention such as oral contraceptives or tamoxifen. However, prophylactic removal of the breasts and ovaries is not 100% protective.

Reliance on genetic testing as predictors of breast and ovarian cancer is not scientifically supported. Analysis of family history, especially multiple affected first- and second-degree relatives, both maternal and paternal, with early onset of disease is the cornerstone of risk assessment. Identifying the precise mutation in a single affected relative makes it easier to look for the same mutation in other family members. BRCA 1 and BRCA 2 analysis should begin with investigation of the affected family member.

RELATIVE RISK (RR)

It is important to remember that while a relative risk greater than 1 may be mathematically correct, unless the relative risk exceeds 2:1 there is only a weak epidemiological association between the risk factor and disease. Clinical decisions should not be overly influenced unless the relative risk is greater than 2:1. Physicians have for years dealt with the risk of unopposed estrogens causing endometrial cancer. By comparison, the relative risk of unopposed estrogen causing endometrial cancer is 5:1. This is far greater than most risk factors for breast cancer and yet the majority of women who take unopposed estrogen do not develop endometrial cancer. Family history of breast cancer increases the patient's relative risk, which increases further if the patient's relative was premenopausal at the time of diagnosis or had bilateral disease (Table 8.2)[2]. Family history is most significant if the relationship is first-degree (i.e. mother, sister or daughter) (Table 8.3)[3]. The risk from a father or brother affected with breast cancer is not well understood.

REFERENCES

1. American Cancer Society, Inc. *Breast Cancer Facts and Figures 2001–2002*. Atlanta: ACS, 2003. Available at http://www.cancer.org/docroot/STT/content/ STT_1x_Breast_Cancer_Facts_and_Figures_2001- 2002.asp. Accessed March 2003
2. Harris JR, Lippman ME, Morrow M, Hellman S. Breast disorders. In Schnitt SJ, Connolly JL, eds. *Diseases of the Breast*. Philadelphia: Lippincott-Raven, 1996
3. Hindle WH, ed. *Breast Care*. New York: Springer Verlag, 1999

SUGGESTED READING

1. Breast-Ovarian Cancer Screening, ACOG Committee Opinion, The American College of Obstetricians and Gynecologist, #239:August 2000
2. Hall JA. *Breast Disorders: Obstetrics and Gynecology Principles and Practice*. Ling FW, Duff P, eds. New York: McGraw-Hill, 2001:938–54

Table 8.3 Effect of positive family history of breast cancer on relative risk (RR). Reproduced with permission from reference 3

First-degree relative affected	Patient's relative risk
Premenopausal	
unilateral	1.8
bilateral	8.8
Postmenopausal	
unilateral	1.2
bilateral	4.0
Aunt or grandmother	1.5
Mother and sister	14.0

KEY POINTS: MALIGNANT BREAST DISEASE RISK FACTORS

1. Only 30% of women with breast cancer have a risk factor other than age or gender
2. The risk of breast cancer advances with age
3. The presence or absence of risk factors should not influence the evaluation of a breast complaint nor the interpretation of results
4. Genetic testing of *BRCA 1* and *BRCA 2* has limited clinical application and firm guidelines for positive results are lacking
5. Most benign conditions do not increase the risk of breast cancer

CHAPTER 9

Benign breast complaints

Although the fear of cancer is usually the motivating factor for a woman to seek healthcare concerning a breast complaint, the vast majority of breast problems arise from benign etiologies. Reassurance may be the only therapy needed in cases such as breast pain (mastalgia). The frequent need for further evaluation, including surgery for mammographic abnormalities, may cause some women to avoid surveillance as they lose faith in the system and wish to eliminate cost, worry, and inconvenience. Primary care physicians and specialists need to do everything possible to keep the patient aware that all concerns need to be investigated and that mammographic screening saves lives. Prompt investigation of all problems, especially mammographic abnormalities, will provide the best opportunity for early diagnosis of cancer.

MASTITIS

Mastitis is an infection of the breast which is usually associated with pregnancy or lactation. The treatment goal is early clinical diagnosis and prompt initiation of antibiotics. Drainage of any abscess should be carried out immediately. Single or serial needle aspirations may successfully drain an abscess and avoid a scar. Incision and drain placement should be carried out promptly if there is not rapid improvement with needle drainage.

Breast feeding may continue although sores on the nipple must be allowed to heal. Mastitis in non-puerperal or older patients is uncommon and the possibility of a tumor or inflammatory carcinoma should be considered.

MASTALGIA

Breast pain or tenderness is a common complaint of women and nearly all women will have mastalgia at some point during their lifetime. Mastalgia may be constant, but it is more usually cyclical with the worst pain just before menstruation as estrogen levels peak. There is no universal agreement as to the etiology of mastalgia and even less agreement as to what is the most effective treatment (Figure 9.1). Reports of caffeine-induced mastalgia have not been scientifically validated although some patients are convinced that reduction of caffeine intake is helpful.

The evaluation of mastalgia requires a careful history and physical examination. The cause may not originate in the breasts but from the chest wall or muscular discomfort. Mammography is indicated if neoplasm is suspected. While breast cancer is usually painless, the presence of tenderness cannot be used to exclude malignancy. A palpable mass or mammogram abnormality should be promptly investigated.

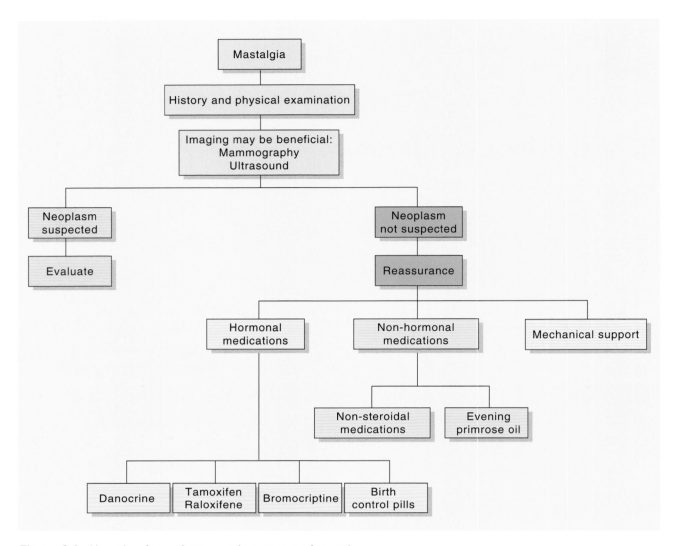

Figure 9.1 Algorithm for evaluation and treatment of mastalgia

When neoplasm is not suspected, the patient may be offered various treatment options. Local measures include a good supporting bra without an underwire apparatus. Medical management includes use of non-steroidal analgesics, or evening primrose oil tablets. Hormonal options should be reserved for severe cases and include danocrine, oral contraceptives, bromocriptine, and selective estrogen receptor modulators such as tamoxifen or raloxifene. Postmenopausal women may experience mastalgia from estrogen replacement therapy and this will usually improve over time or with a lowered dose.

FIBROCYSTIC CHANGES

There is no such entity as fibrocystic breast 'disease' and the term is commonly used to describe lumpy or tender breasts. Fibrocystic change is a physiologic but exaggerated response to estrogen and exists to some degree in all women. Classic symptoms are premenstrual cyclic engorgement with increased breast density which usually minimizes in the proliferative phase of the cycle. A high percentage of breast biopsy specimens have areas of fibrocystic change but are not part of a pathologic process. Fibrocystic breast changes may result in significant tenderness or a palpable mass. The usual clinical finding is an asymmetric lumpy area of the breast which is most commonly in the upper outer quadrant. Unilateral nipple discharge may occasionally be noted. Most fibrocystic areas resolve over a few menstrual cycles without any therapy. The malignant risk of fibrocystic change has been heavily debated and it is felt that there is no increased risk of malignancy in the absence of a significant degree of epithelial proliferation or ductal atypia.

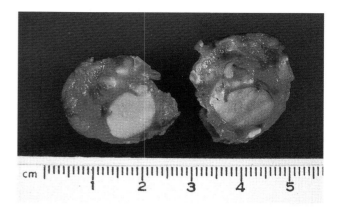

Figure 9.2 Gross specimen: duct ectasia

DUCT ECTASIA

Duct ectasia usually presents with multiple duct nipple discharge and subareolar pain, itching, or burning. A mass or swelling may be palpated under the areola (Figures 9.2 and 9.3). Duct ectasia results from periductal inflammation leading to fibrosis and dilatation of the duct. Rupture of the duct may occur and can result in inflammation and fat necrosis. Excision of the involved duct is required for treatment and to rule out carcinoma.

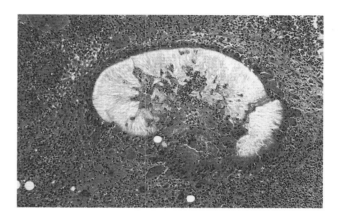

Figure 9.3 Histology: duct ectasia

FAT NECROSIS

Patients with fat necrosis present with a tender ill-defined mass. Mammography may suggest malignant changes with microcalcifications and a stellate mass. Fat necrosis will usually originate from trauma although the patient may not be aware of when the injury took place. A poorly-fitted bra, especially the underwired type, may lead to fat necrosis and result in a ridge along the inferior margin of the breast. There is no malignant potential although excisional biopsy may be required to establish the diagnosis.

FIBROADENOMA

Fibroadenoma is the most common breast neoplasm. Fibroadenomas are benign and do not increase the patient's subsequent risk for breast cancer. The nodules are firm, rubbery, and circumscribed. They often present in adolescents or women in their twenties. Fibroadenomas are painless and do not change size in relation to the menstrual cycle. Twenty percent of women with fibroadenoma have more than one nodule either at the time of diagnosis or at a later age. Approximately one-third of fibroadenomas will regress in size or disappear when followed over time. Fibroadenomas may be electively removed or followed clinically if the diagnosis has been confirmed through agreement of the results of clinical examination, mammography, and fine needle aspiration cytology (or needle biopsy).

BENIGN BREAST DISEASE AND MALIGNANT RISK

Benign breast disease often makes patients concerned that they may have an increased risk of breast cancer. It is important to stress to the patient her real risk, as out-of-date information and misguided rumors may create needless concern. As recently as just a few years ago, trauma was thought to increase the risk of breast cancer. Nonproliferative disorders such as cysts, fibrocystic changes, mild hyperplasia, and fibroadenoma result in no increased risk of breast cancer. Proliferative lesions without atypia result in a slightly increased risk. A significantly increased risk results from the proliferative lesions with atypia, such as atypical ductal hyperplasia, atypical lobular hyperplasia, and lobular carcinoma *in situ* (Table 9.1).

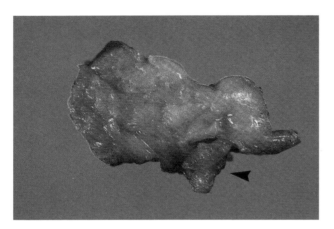

Figure 9.4 Benign breast intraductal papilloma: gross specimen. Intraductal papilloma usually presents with unilateral single duct nipple discharge that is often a green/black color or bloody. Papillomas are usually benign but require removal for diagnosis

Table 9.1 Benign breast conditions and relative risk of cancer

No increased risk
    adenosis
    cysts
    fibroadenoma
    ductal ectasia
    mild hyperplasia
    fibrosis
    mastitis
    trauma

Slightly increased risk (1.5–2 times)
    hyperplasia: moderate, florid, solid, or papillary
    papilloma

Moderately increased risk (3–5 times)
    atypical hyperplasia, ductal or lobular
    lobular carcinoma *in situ*

KEY POINTS: BENIGN BREAST COMPLAINTS

1. Most benign conditions do not increase the risk of breast cancer
2. Atypical hyperplasia increases the risk of breast cancer three- to fivefold
3. Breast tenderness or mastalgia rarely originates from breast cancer and may originate from the chest wall
4. Mastalgia usually resolves after reassurance that the patient does not have cancer
5. Fibroadenoma is a benign breast tumor that can be observed or electively removed once the diagnosis is secure

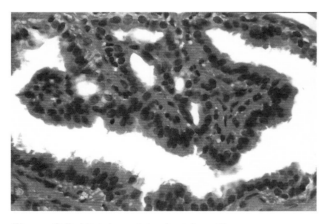

Figure 9.5 Histology: intraductal papilloma

CHAPTER 10

Galactorrhea and pathologic nipple discharge

Ten percent of non-puerperal women experience spontaneous nipple discharge and approximately 80% of these can express secretions. Nipple discharge is differentiated into either galactorrhea or pathologic nipple discharge (PND). The diagnosis of galactorrhea or PND can be made on the basis of the history and physical examination (Figure 10.1)[1].

Galactorrhea results from elevated prolactin levels and is usually induced, bilateral, and from multiple duct openings on the nipple. Galactorrhea secretion is watery or milky and does not contain blood or pus. PND results from a problem within the breast and is spontaneous, unilateral, and from a single duct opening on the nipple. The secretion is bloody, serous, serosanguineous, or watery. The most common cause of PND is a benign papilloma (35–48% of cases). Duct ectasia (17–36%) is the next most likely cause and results from a benign inflammatory condition of the duct wall. Carcinoma is the least likely cause of PND (5–21% of cases)[2].

Knowledge of breast anatomy will help locate the origin of the cause of PND. Each lobe has its own unique terminal or excretory duct, therefore knowing the location of the duct opening will relate to the location of the abnormality in the respective breast.

Galactorrhea results from the lactogenic effect of increased serum prolactin levels. Table 10.1 lists

Table 10.1 Effect of medications on prolactin secretion

Inhibition
    dopamine
    L-dopa
Stimulation
Psychotropics
    phenothiazines
    tricyclic antidepressants
    opiates
    SSRI antidepressants
Hormones
    estrogen
    thyrotropin-releasing hormone
Antihypertensives
    methyldopa
    reserpine
    verapamil
Antiemetics
    sulpiride
    metoclopramide
Anesthetics
H_2 receptor antagonists
    cimetidine

the effect of various medications on prolactin secretion. Prolactin synthesis from the pituitary gland is controlled by central nervous system neurotransmitters from the hypothalamus. Dopamine, a prolactin inhibiting factor (PIF), is the major inhibitor of prolactin release. A specific hypothalamic

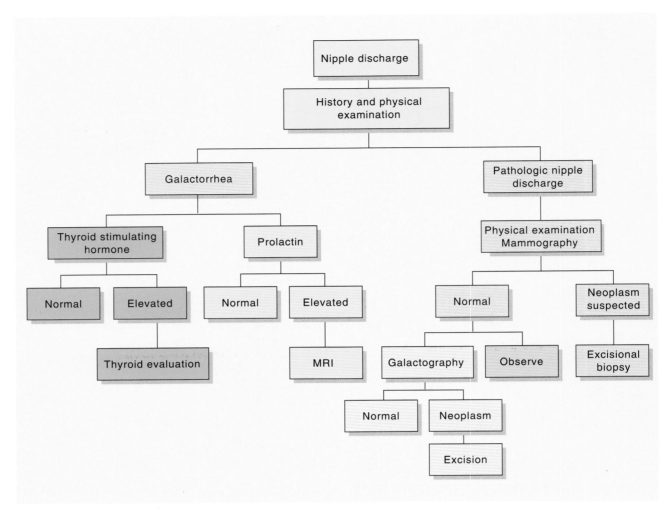

Figure 10.1 Algorithm for evaluation of nipple discharge. Figure reproduced with permission from Hall JA. Galactorrhea and nipple discharge. In Stovall TG, Ling FW, eds. *Gynecology for the Primary Care Physician*. Philadelphia: Current Medicine, 1995; 5–10

prolactin releasing factor has not been isolated. Both serotonin and thyrotropin-releasing factor stimulate prolactin release. Serotonin is thought to be the primary prolactin releasing factor as thyrotropin releasing factor stimulates only minimally. Hyperprolactinemia may be difficult to diagnose because nearly two-thirds of women with elevated prolactin levels do not have galactorrhea. Estrogen suppresses the hypothalamus resulting in lower production of PIF and thus increased levels of prolactin. The effect of estrogen on the hypothalamus results in increased levels of prolactin at puberty and during the third trimester of pregnancy.

Estrogen also inhibits the action of prolactin on the breast and thus lactation usually does not occur during pregnancy even though prolactin levels may reach 200ng/ml during the third trimester. The local action of estrogen also inhibits galactorrhea in women using estrogen hormonal products such as oral contraceptive pills.

TREATMENT

PND is treated surgically once investigation reveals the location of the problem within the breast (Figure 10.2). Treatment of galactorrhea

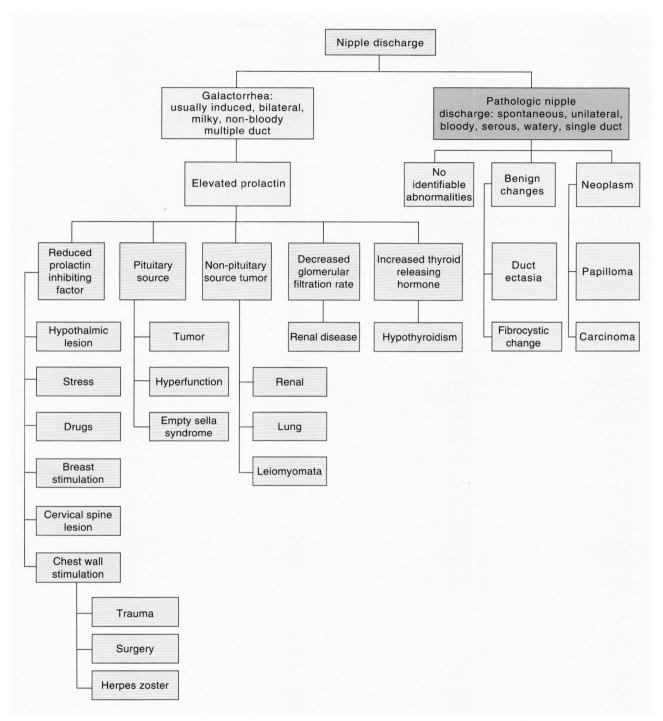

Figure 10.2 Etiology of nipple discharge. Figure reproduced with permission from Hall JA. Galactorrhea and nipple discharge. In Stovall TG, Ling FW, eds. *Gynecology for the Primary Care Physician*. Philadelphia: Current Medicine, 1995

depends on the patient's diagnosis and tolerance to the secretions. Alteration of medications or decreased breast stimulation may return prolactin levels to normal. Women with functional hyperprolactinemia, empty sella syndrome, or microadenoma who do not wish to conceive or are not concerned by the secretion do not require treatment and should be followed clinically with serial prolactin levels. Headaches, visual changes, or prolactin levels over 100 ng/ml increase the likelihood of a sellar or suprasellar tumor. Fortunately most microadenomas (less than 1 cm) rarely enlarge and many regress over time. Pregnancy, oral contraceptives, and hormonal replacement therapy do not stimulate growth and are not contraindicated. Induced estrogen deficiency from hyperprolactinemia may increase the risk of osteoporosis. Non-lactitroph pituitary tumors or other central nervous system disorders will require referral. Microadenomas are treated with dopamine agonists and rarely require surgery. Macroadenomas (1 cm or larger) are also treated with dopamine agonists. Surgery is reserved for those who fail to respond to therapy or have clinical problems such as persistent headaches or visual field loss.

Recurrence of hyperprolactinemia and tumor growth is not uncommon after surgical resection. Serial prolactin levels and MRI scans may be necessary to follow patients on therapy for pituitary adenomas. Half of all pituitary macroadenomas treated with the dopamine agonist bromocriptine will regress in size by 50% and another quarter will reduce by 30%. Long-term treatment is usually required for macroadenomas as nearly 60% of patients experience tumor regrowth after discontinuation of bromocriptine. Medical therapy is usually discontinued after conception but may be required during pregnancy if there is significant sized tumor causing headaches or visual field changes. Breastfeeding is not contraindicated with either micro- or macroadenomas.

REFERENCES

1. Hall JA. Galactorrhea and nipple discharge. In Stovall TG, Ling FW, eds. *Gynecology for the Primary Care Physician*. Philadelphia: Current Medicine, 1995; 5–10
2. Heshlag A, Peterson LM. Endocrine disorders. In Berek J, Adashi E, Hillard P, eds. *Novak's Gynecology*. Baltimore: Williams and Wilkins, 1996:833–64

KEY POINTS: GALACTORRHEA AND PATHOLOGIC NIPPLE DISCHARGE

1. Galactorrhea results from elevated prolactin levels and the lactogenic effect on the breast and not from intrinsic disease
2. Pathologic nipple discharge results from a disease process from a specific location within the breast
3. Carcinoma is the least likely cause of pathologic nipple discharge
4. The differentiation between galactorrhea and pathologic nipple secretion is possible based on history and physical examination
5. Prolactinomas are treated medically and rarely require surgery

CHAPTER 11

Breast cancer surgery

OVERVIEW

For treatment purposes, breast cancer may be divided into:

(1) Stage 0: non-invasive carcinoma, primarily duct cell carcinoma *in situ* (DCIS) and lobular carcinoma *in situ* (LCIS)

(2) Stage I, II, some IIIA

(3) Some Stage IIIA, IIIB: inoperable locoregional invasive carcinoma

(4) Stage IV: metastatic/recurrent breast carcinoma

In 2002, the American Joint Committee on Cancer (AJCC) updated their staging system for breast cancer (see Appendix). Beyond staging, biological factors including age, menopausal status, involvement of axilliary lymph nodes, hormones (estrogen and progesterone) receptor status, growth phase of cancer cells, oncogene expression, and other information, provide prognostic information for survival in breast cancer patients.

DUCTAL CELL CARCINOMA *IN SITU*

Patient with limited DCIS, in whom negative margins are achieved by initial excision (lumpectomy) or by re-excision, are usually offered ipsilateral breast irradiation as initial therapy. Total mastectomy is a treatment option. Axillary dissection is not recommended for patients undergoing lumpectomy or mastectomy for DCIS. Patients with widespread DCIS are treated with total mastectomy without lymph node sampling. Women treated with mastectomy for DCIS are appropriate candidates for breast reconstruction.

Patients undergoing breast conserving therapy for DCIS are given tamoxifen treatment after completion of radiation therapy. Tamoxifen treatment is intended to decrease the development/ reduce the risk of ipsilateral breast recurrence and development of a contralateral second primary breast cancer.

LOBULAR CARCINOMA *IN SITU*

Observation alone is the preferred option for women diagnosed with lobular carcinoma *in situ* (LCIS), with the risk of developing invasive carcinoma being low (approximately 21% over 15 years). The risk of an invasive breast cancer, following a diagnosis of LCIS, is equal in both breasts. LCIS can be treated with bilateral mastectomy to minimize future risk. These women are appropriate candidates for breast reconstruction. Treated LCIS patients who have been given tamoxifen for 5 years have an approximately 56% reduction in the risk of developing invasive breast cancer.

TREATMENT OF EARLY STAGE BREAST CANCER (STAGES I, IIA & IIB)

Randomized trials have documented the equivalence of breast conserving therapy with lumpectomy, axillary dissection and breast irradiation to mastectomy with axillary lymph node dissection in women with Stage I and II breast cancer (Figure 11.1). Relative contraindications to breast conserving therapy include prior radiotherapy to the breast or chest wall, positive breast biopsy margins (lumpectomy, re-excision), multicentric disease, most multifocal disease and pre-existing connective tissue disease, other than rheumatoid arthritis (Table 11.1).

Histopathologic assessment of the axillary lymph nodes becomes more conservative with transition from Levels I and II lymph nodes to sampling Level I lymph nodes to sentinel lymph node biopsy. In appropriate women, the sentinel lymph node biopsy is a less invasive alternative to axillary lymph node dissection. Sentinel lymph node biopsy involves injection of blue dye and/or radioisotope in the

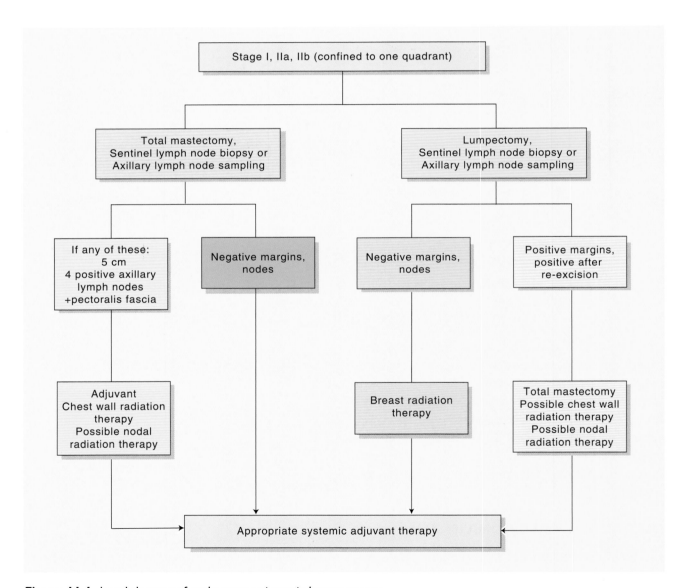

Figure 11.1 Local therapy of early-stage unicentric breast cancer

Table 11.1 Breast conservation considerations

Ideal candidate
Small, single tumor (< 4–5 cm)
Clear surgical margins
Cosmetically acceptable result expected
Multidisciplinary/patient agreement

Features that may compromise breast conservation treatment
Multifocal/multicentric disease
Inability to achieve negative surgical margins
Extensive intraductal component
Extensive disease – associated microcalcifications on mammography
Pregnant patient
Previous radiation therapy to same breast
Significant collagen vascular disease
Multidisciplinary/patient disagreement

periareolar, peritumoral or subcutaneous tissue of the affected breast. Following isolation and excision, the sentinel lymph node is closely examined. It is proven to be more predictive of axillary lymph node metastasis status than any other tumor prognostic factor. Studies indicate that adjacent non-sentinel lymph nodes are very rarely involved if the sentinel lymph node is tumor free. Sentinel lymph node biopsy alone is emerging as the gold standard of care treatment for most clinically node-negative women with early breast cancer.

RADIATION THERAPY

Patients with early invasive breast cancer treated with lumpectomy and lymph node sampling receive ipsilateral whole-breast radiation in order to decrease the recurrence rate. Similarly, patients treated with mastectomy who have tumors greater than 5 cm in greatest diameter or positive surgical margins are at sufficiently high risk per local recurrence to warrant postmastectomy radial therapy to the chest wall.

SYSTEMIC ADJUVANT THERAPY

Small tumors (up to 0.5 cm in greatest diameter) with negative lymph nodes are generally not candidates for adjuvant systemic therapy. Patients with tumors 0.6–1 cm in diameter with negative lymph nodes are divided into low or high risk groups by using prognostic features such as lymph–vascular space invasion, high nuclear grade, high growth phase fraction and oncogene overexpression. Patients with tumors greater than 1 cm in greatest diameter or positive lymph nodes are appropriate candidates for adjuvant systemic therapy. Chemotherapy regimens used in systemic adjuvant therapy are individualized.

Tamoxifen therapy is utilized in estrogen receptor positive patients as an alternative to, or following, systemic chemotherapy for ipsilateral and contralateral (lumpectomy patients), or contralateral (mastectomy patients) breast cancer risk reduction.

KEY POINTS: BREAST CANCER SURGERY

1. Surgical technique options must be integrated into a multidisciplinary approach for women with newly diagnosed breast cancer
2. Breast conservatism is the preferred option for most women with small, newly diagnosed breast tumors (see Table 11.1)
3. Complete surgical excision of the malignant lesion with clear margins is the intent of a breast lumpectomy
4. Controversy exists surrounding the extent of surgery necessary for the recovery of axillary lymph nodes in patients with invasive breast cancer. Ipsilateral axillary lymphadenectomy, lymph node sampling or sentinel lymph node excision are options individualized by patient
5. Modified radical mastectomy (breast and axillary lymph nodes) remains an option to lumpectomy/ lymph node sampling in patients with early breast cancer or those less than ideal candidates for lumpectomy (see Table 11.1)

CHAPTER 12

Hormone replacement therapy and breast disease

Despite over 50 epidemiological studies and at least 10 meta-analyses over the past 25 years, the association between estrogen replacement therapy (ERT) and breast cancer remains controversial[1]. Until the first report of the Women's Health Initiative (WHI) clinical trial was published[2], a pooled analysis of 90% of the international data on breast cancer and hormone replacement therapy (HRT) indicated a small likelihood of there being a direct association[3].

While the WHI report has had a profound influence on HRT, particularly regarding the breast cancer risk, a critical review of the WHI data is appropriate to assist the clinician in individualizing patient care. The WHI was intended to be a randomized controlled primary prevention trial

examining the risk and benefits of combined HRT. From 1993 to 1998, 16 608 out of a planned 19 000 postmenopausal women aged 50 to 79 years were recruited. Study criteria included an intact uterus; and participants were randomly assigned to receive 0.625 mg conjugated equine estrogen plus 2.5 mg medroxyprogesterone acetate daily. Women with severe menopausal symptoms were excluded. The primary outcome was coronary heart disease with invasive breast cancer as the primary adverse outcome. Secondary study points included stroke, deep vein thrombophlebitis or pulmonary embolism, bone fractures, colon cancer and endometrial cancer.

After a mean of 5.2 years of follow-up, the study Data and Safety Monitoring Board stopped

Table 12.1 Relative and absolute risk or benefit seen in estrogen plus progestin arm of the Women's Health Initiative (n = 16 608, placebo and study drug). Table adapted with permission from Rossouw JE, Anderson GL, Prentice RL, et al. Risks and benefits of estrogen plus progestin in healthy postmenopausal women: principal results from the Women's Health Initiative randomized controlled trial. J Am Med Assoc 2002;288:321–33

Health event	Relative risk vs. placebo group at 5.2 years	Increased absolute risk per 10 000 women/year	Increased absolute benefit per 10 000 women/year
Heart attacks	1.29	7	
Strokes	1.41	8	
Breast cancer	1.26	8	
Thromboembolic events	2.11	18	
Colorectal cancer	0.63		6
Hip fractures	0.66		5

the estrogen plus progestin trial arm because of a predetermined incidence of invasive breast cancer (but not a statistically significant increased risk).

Discontinuation of the estrogen plus progestin arm of the trial was based on data that demonstrated a hazard ratio of 1.26 (95% confidence interval, hazard ratio of 0.83–1.92 with adjusted 95% CI). The estrogen-only arm of the study was not discontinued and is scheduled to conclude in 2005. The WHI study demonstrated increased risk of heart attacks, strokes, thromboembolic events and breast cancer. Benefit was demonstrated in reduction of colorectal cancer and hip fractures (see Table 12.1).

Also in 2002, Weiss and colleagues[4] reported a large, multicenter, population-based, case–control study designed to examine the relationship of HRT and breast cancer risk based on regimen, duration and recency of use. They demonstrated that 5 or more years of continuous combined HRT was associated with an increased breast cancer risk (1.45, 95% CI). The authors noted that breast cancer risk dissipated after HRT was discontinued. They also noted that progesterone administered in an uninterrupted regimen may be a contributing factor and there is no positive association between breast cancer risk and HRT regimens, other than the continuous combined method.

Since its publication in July 2002, the WHI study has been heralded as having changed HRT administration forever. The US Food and Drug Administration (FDA) initiated warning labels on estrogen–progesterone packaging and the US Preventative Services Task Force (USPSTF) issued new recommendations regarding HRT.

Goodman and colleagues[5] have critiqued the WHI results based on the study design, in particular randomization, blinding, and drop-out rates appropriate to this discussion. They note that the premature discontinuation of the estrogen plus progesterone arm of the WHI study means that the calculated power of the statistical evaluation is lost, and that all conclusions stated by the authors must be critically evaluated. Further, they conclude that if the study does not meet the

predetermined power and statistical significance, including the number of continuous participants and years of follow-up, then the study is flawed and may be invalid. Specific issues raised by the Goodman *et al.* review include:

(1) Excluding women with severe menopausal symptoms resulted in a majority of women who were receiving estrogen and progesterone therapy being more than 10 years postmenopausal, resulting in some degree of pre-existing atherosclerosis. The beneficial effect of hormone therapy on the cardiovascular system would be diminished in the presence of already existent atherosclerosis and this could account for a nominal increase in cardiac events. This population may not represent the typical early menopausal patient group presenting with quality-of-life symptoms. Nor was the WHI study sensitive enough to identify subclinical coronary disease or disease progression.

(2) The absent rates of coronary disease, stroke, pulmonary embolus and breast-on end points per 10 000 women-years were marginally significant. There were a combined total of 358 heart attacks, strokes, deep vein thromboses, osteoporotic fractures and breast cancers. There were 583 women completely lost to follow-up. More women were lost to follow-up than had 'end-point events'.

(3) The WHI had a substantial dropout rate of approximately 40% for both placebo and the estrogen plus progesterone groups. A greater than 20% dropout rate in any study usually initiates a thorough analysis of the event.

(4) The effect of unblinding 3444 women in the study group is critical. Forty percent of the treatment group was unblinded but only 6.7% of the placebo group was. Unblinding occurred primarily because of excessive vaginal bleeding. A bias could have been introduced as any departure from the study treatment protocol reduces the chances of finding a treatment difference.

(5) A positive beneficial effect of estrogen plus progesterone on fracture rate and colon cancer was demonstrated. This is the first time that

protection against colon cancer – the third most common cancer in the world – has been demonstrated prospectively.

(6) Conclusions drawn from increased invasive breast cancer risk data, with confidence intervals that do not support statistical significance, do not seem to be justified as the differences could have occurred by random chance. The incidents of breast cancer increases in years 4 and 5 of the study could support an explanation of estrogen plus progesterone therapy activation of pre-existing breast malignancy. The short duration of the study makes it unlikely that the cancers started after hormone therapy was initiated.

In conclusion, many of the differences shown in the WHI study between the estrogen plus progesterone group and the control group could have occurred by random chance alone in this older group of women. Bias and confounding could have further affected the reported results. Quality-of-life benefits of HRT, inclusion of younger menopausal women, and the short duration of the study should induce the clinician to individualize the potential short- and long-term benefits to each individual patient based on her personal risk profile.

OTHER IMPORTANT HORMONE REPLACEMENT AND BREAST CANCER ISSUES

Several other important issues regarding HRT and breast cancer are worthy of notation. Estrogen replacement therapy taken at the time of breast cancer diagnosis does not increase either the risk of recurrence or death in patients with early breast cancer[6–8].

The possible benefits of HRT for breast cancer patients taking tamoxifen have been considered[9]. The combined use of tamoxifen and HRT appears to reduce the risk and side-effects of each agent. Compliance with tamoxifen use appears to be increased in patients simultaneously taking HRT. This information provides the background for ongoing and future studies to consider the use of this treatment option in breast cancer patients.

REFERENCES

1. Bush TL, Whiteman M, Flaws JA. Hormone replacement therapy and breast cancer: a qualitative review. *Obstet Gynecol* 2001;98:498–508
2. Writing Group for the Women's Health Initiative Investigators. Risk and benefits of estrogen plus progesterone in healthy postmenopausal women. *J Am Med Assoc* 2002;288:321–33
3. Collaborative Group on Hormone Factors in Breast Cancer and Hormone Replacement Therapy. *Lancet* 1997;350:10947–59
4. Weiss LK, Burkman RT, Cushing-Haugen KL, *et al.* Hormone replacement therapy regimens and breast cancer risk. *Obstet Gynecol* 2002;100:1148–58
5. Goodman N, Goldzieher J, Ayala C. Critique of the report from the Writing Group of the WHI. *Menopausal Med* 2003;10:1–4
6. O'Meara ES, Rossing MA, Daling Jr, *et al.* Hormone replacement therapy after diagnosis of breast cancer in relation to recurrence and mortality. *J Natl Cancer Inst* 2001;93:754–62
7. Nandra K, Bastian LA, Schulz K. Hormone replacement therapy and the risk of death from breast cancer. *Am J Obstet Gynecol* 2002;186:325–34
8. Natrajam P, Gambrell RD. Estrogen replacement therapy in patients with early breast cancer. *Am J Obstet Gynecol* 2002;187:289–95
9. Bowanni B, Gonzaga AG, Romensz N. Hormonal therapy and chemoprevention. *Breast J* 2000;6:5: 317–23

KEY POINTS: HRT AND BREAST DISEASE

1. Good epidemiologic evidence exists demonstrating the benefit of HRT on a patient's osteoporosis, cardiovascular disease, and genitourinary symptoms and also shows that it has the potential to lengthen life
2. Simultaneously, a meta-analysis of 90% of the international literature on oral HRT has shown an associated small increase of breast cancer (relative risk 1.14, $p = 0.00001$)
3. Chemoprevention with tamoxifen in patients at high risk for breast cancer should be determined by objective calculation of actual risk (modified Gail model)
4. Low-dose HRT is an option for patients following treatment of *in situ* or early invasive breast cancer

APPENDIX

The American Joint Committee on Cancer's Staging Form for Breast Cancer. Used with the permission of the American Joint Committee on Cancer (AJCC), Chicago, Illinois. The original source for this material is the *AJCC Cancer Staging Manual, Sixth Edition* (2002) published by Springer-Verlag New York, www.springer-ny.com

BREAST	
Hospital Name/Address	**Patient Name/Information**

Type of Specimen _____ Histopathologic Type _____

Tumor Size _____ Laterality: ☐ Bilateral ☐ Left ☐ Right

DEFINITIONS

Clinical	Pathologic		Primary Tumor (T)
☐	☐	TX	Primary tumor cannot be assessed
☐	☐	TO	No evidence of primary tumor
☐	☐	Tis	Carcinoma *in situ*
☐	☐	Tis	(DCIS) Ductal carcinoma *in situ*
☐	☐	Tis	(LCIS) Lobular carcinoma *in situ*
☐	☐	Tis	(Paget's) Paget's disease of the nipple with no tumor *Note:* Paget's disease associated with a tumor is classified according to the size of the tumor.
☐	☐	T1	Tumor 2 cm or less in greatest dimension
☐	☐	T1mic	Microinvasion 0.1 cm or less in greatest dimension
☐	☐	T1a	Tumor more than 0.1 cm but not more than 0.5 cm in greatest dimension
☐	☐	T1b	Tumor more than 0.5 cm but not more than 1 cm in greatest dimension
☐	☐	T1c	Tumor more than 1 cm but not more than 2 cm in greatest dimension
☐	☐	T2	Tumor more than 2 cm but not more than 5 cm in greatest dimension
☐	☐	T3	Tumor more than 5 cm in greatest dimension
☐	☐	T4	Tumor of any size with direct extension to (a) chest wall or (b) skin, only as described below.
☐	☐	T4a	Extension to chest wall, not including pectoralis muscle
☐	☐	T4b	Edema (including peau d'orange) or ulceration of the skin of the breast, or satellite skin nodules confined to the same breast
☐	☐	T4c	Both T4a and T4b
☐	☐	T4d	Inflammatory carcinoma

Notes

1. *Clinically apparent* is defined as detected by imaging studies (excluding lymphoscintigraphy) or by clinical examination.
2. Classification is based on axillary lymph node dissection with or without sentinel lymph node dissection. Classification based solely on sentinel lymph node dissection without subsequent axillary lymph node dissection is designated (sn) for "sentinel node," e.g., pNO(i+)(sn).
3. Isolated tumor cells (ITC) are defined as single tumor cells or small cell clusters not greater than 0.2 mm, usually detected only by immunohistochemical (IHC) or molecular methods but which may be verified on H&E stains. ITCs do not usually show evidence of metastatic activity (e.g., proliferation or stromal reaction.)
4. RT-PCR: reverse transcriptase/polymerase chain reaction.
5. *Not clinically apparent* is defined as not detected by imaging studies (excluding lymphoscintigraphy) or by clinical examination.
6. If associated with greater than 3 positive axillary lymph nodes, the internal mammary nodes are classified as pN3b to reflect increased tumor burden.
7. T1 includes T1mic

(continued over)

BREAST

Clinical	Regional Lymph Nodes (N)

☐ NX — Regional lymph nodes cannot be assessed (e.g., previously removed)

☐ N0 — No regional lymph node metastasis

☐ N1 — Metastasis in movable ipsilateral axillary lymph node(s)

☐ N2 — Metastases in ipsilateral axillary lymph nodes fixed or matted, or in clinically apparent[1] ipsilateral internal mammary nodes in the *absence* of clinically evident axillary lymph node metastasis

☐ N2a — Metastasis in ipsilateral axillary lymph nodes fixed to one another (matted) or to other structures

☐ N2b — Metastases only in clinically apparent[1] ipsilateral internal mammary nodes and in the *absence* of clinically evident axillary lymph node metastasis

☐ N3 — Metastasis in ipsilateral infraclavicular lymph node(s) with or without axillary lymph node involvement, or in clinically apparent[1] ipsilateral internal mammary lymph node(s) and in the *presence* of clinically evident axillary lymph node metastasis; or metastasis in ipsilateral supraclavicular lymph node(s) with or without axillary or internal mammary lymph node involvement

☐ N3a — Metastasis in ipsilateral infraclavicular lymph node(s) and axillary lymph node(s)

☐ N3b — Metastasis in ipsilateral internal mammary lymph node(s) and axillary lymph node(s)

☐ N3c — Metastasis in ipsilateral supraclavicular lymph node(s)

Pathologic	Regional Lymph Nodes (pN)[2]

☐ pNX — Regional lymph nodes cannot be assessed (e.g., previously removed, or not removed for pathologic study)

☐ pN0 — No regional lymph node metastasis histologically, no additional examination for isolated tumor cells (ITC)[3]

☐ pN0(i⁻) — No regional lymph node metastasis histologically, negative IHC

☐ pN0(i+) — No regional lymph node metastasis histologically, positive IHC, no IHC cluster greater than 0.2 mm

☐ pN0(mol⁻) — No regional lymph node metastasis histologically, negative molecular findings (RT-PCR)[4]

☐ pN0(mol+) — No regional lymph node metastasis histologically, positive molecular findings (RT-PCR)[4]

☐ pN1 — Metastasis in 1 to 3 axillary lymph nodes, and/or in internal mammary nodes with microscopic disease detected by sentinel lymph node dissection but not clinically apparent[5]

☐ pN1mi — Micrometastasis (greater than 0.2 mm, none greater than 2.0 mm)

☐ pN1a — Metastasis in 1 to 3 axillary lymph nodes

☐ pN1b — Metastasis in internal mammary nodes with microscopic disease detected by sentinel lymph node dissection but not clinically apparent[5]

☐ pN1c — Metastasis in 1 to 3 axillary lymph nodes and in internal mammary lymph nodes with microscopic disease detected by sentinel lymph node dissection but not clinically apparent[5,6]

☐ pN2 — Metastasis in 4 to 9 axillary lymph nodes, or in clinically apparent[1] internal mammary lymph nodes in the *absence* of axillary lymph node metastasis

☐ pN2a — Metastasis in 4 to 9 axillary lymph nodes (at least one tumor deposit greater than 2.0 mm)

☐ pN2b — Metastasis in clinically apparent[1] internal mammary lymph nodes in the *absence* of axillary lymph node metastasis

☐ pN3 — Metastasis in 10 or more axillary lymph nodes, or in infraclavicular lymph nodes, or in clinically apparent[1] ipsilateral internal mammary lymph nodes in the *presence* of 1 or more positive axillary lymph nodes; or in more than 3 axillary lymph nodes with clinically negative microscopic metastasis in internal mammary lymph nodes; or in ipsilateral supraclavicular lymph nodes

☐ pN3a — Metastasis in 10 or more axillary lymph nodes (at least one tumor deposit greater than 2.0mm), or metastasis to the infraclavicular lymph nodes

☐ pN3b — Metastasis in clinically apparent[1] ipsilateral internal mammary lymph nodes in the *presence* of 1 or more positive axillary lymph nodes; or in more than 3 axillary lymph nodes and in internal mammary lymph nodes with microscopic disease detected by sentinel lymph node dissection but not clinically apparent[5]

☐ pN3c — Metastasis in ipsilateral supraclavicular lymph nodes

BREAST

Clinical	Pathologic	Distant Metastasis (M)
☐	☐	MX Distant metastasis cannot be assessed
☐	☐	M0 No distant metastasis
☐	☐	M1 Distant metastasis

Biopsy of metastatic site performed.... ☐ Y...... ☐ N

Source of pathologic metastatic specimen _____

Stage Grouping

Clinical	Pathologic				
☐	☐	0	Tis	N0	M0
☐	☐	I	T1[7]	N0	M0
☐	☐	IIA	T0	N1	M0
			T1[7]	N1	M0
			T2	N0	M0
☐	☐	IIB	T2	N1	M0
			T3	N0	M0
☐	☐	IIIA	T0	N2	M0
			T1[7]	N2	M0
			T2	N2	M0
			T3	N1	M0
			T3	N2	M0
☐	☐	IIIB	T4	N0	M0
			T4	N1	M0
			T4	N2	M0
☐	☐	IIIC	Any T	N3	M0
☐	☐	IV	Any T	Any N	M1

Note: Stage designation may be changed if post-surgical imaging studies reveal the presence of distant metastases, provided that the studies are carried out within 4 months of diagnosis in the absence of disease progression and provided that the patient has not received neoadjuvant therapy.

Histologic Grade (G)

All invasive breast carcinomas with the exception of medullary carcinoma should be graded. The Nottingham combined histologic grade (Elston-Ellis modification of Scarff-Bloom-Richardson grading system) is recommended. The grade for a tumor is determined by assessing morphologic features (tubule formation, nuclear pleomorphism, and mitotic count), assigning a value of 1 (favorable) to 3 (unfavorable) for each feature, and adding together the scores for all three categories. A combined score of 3–5 points is designated as grade 1; a combined score of 6–7 points is grade 2; a combined score of 8–9 points is grade 3.

Histologic Grade (*Nottingham combined histologic grade is recommended*)

☐ GX   Grade cannot be assessed
☐ G1   Low combined histologic grade (favorable)
☐ G2   Intermediate combined histologic grade (moderately favorable)
☐ G3   High combined histologic grade (unfavorable)

Residual Tumor (R)

☐ RX   Presence of residual tumor cannot be assessed
☐ R0   No residual tumor
☐ R1   Microscopic residual tumor
☐ R2   Macroscopic residual tumor

BREAST

Additional Descriptors

For identification of special cases of TNM or pTNM classifications, the "m" suffix and "y," "r," and "a" prefixes are used. Although they do not affect the stage grouping, they indicate cases needing separate analysis.

m suffix indicates the presence of multiple primary tumors in a single site and is recorded in parentheses: pT(m)NM.

y prefix indicates those cases in which classification is performed during or following initial multi-modality therapy. The cTNM or pTNM category is identified by a "y" prefix. The ycTNM or ypTNM categorizes the extent of tumor actually present at the time of that examination. The "y" categorization is not an estimate of tumor prior to multimodality therapy.

r prefix indicates a recurrent tumor when staged after a disease-free interval, and is identified by the "r" prefix: rTNM.

a prefix designates the stage determined at autopsy: aTNM.

Prognostic indicators (if applicable)

Notes
Additional Descriptors
Lymphatic Vessel Invasion (L)
LX Lymphatic vessel invasion cannot be assessed
L0 No lymphatic vessel invasion
L1 Lymphatic vessel invasion

Venous Invasion (V)
VX Venous invasion cannot be assessed
V0 No venous invasion
V1 Microscopic venous invasion
V2 Macroscopic venous invasion

ILLUSTRATION
Indicate on diagram primary tumor and regional nodes involved.

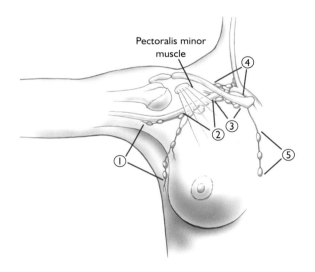

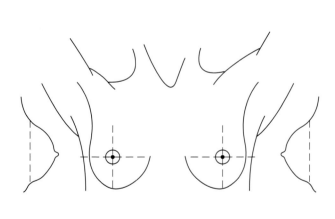

Schematic diagram of breast and regional lymph nodes:
1. Low axillary, Level I
2. Mid-axillary, Level II
3. High axillary, apical, Level III
4. Supraclavicular
5. Internal mammary nodes

Physician's Signature_____ Date _____

Index